GIFTS OF TIME

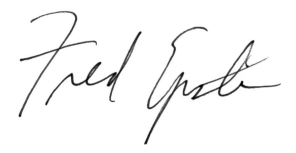

sept 93

With best wishes

Fred Epstein

GIFTS

O F

TIME

Fred J. Epstein, M. D.,
and
Elaine Fantle Shimberg

WILLIAM MORROW AND COMPANY, INC.   NEW YORK

Library of Congress Cataloging-in-Publication Data

Shimberg, Elaine Fantle, 1937–
  Gifts of time / Fred J. Epstein, M.D., and Elaine Fantle Shimberg
      p.   cm.
  ISBN 0-688-11029-0
  1. Epstein, Fred, 1937–   .   2. Neurosurgeons—United States—Biography.
3. Pediatric surgeons—United States—Biography.   4. Brain—Cancer—Patients—
United States.   5. Tumors in children—Patients—United States.   I. Epstein, Fred,
1937–   .   II. Title.
RD592.9.E67S55   1993
617.4'8'092—dc20
  [B]   92-21589
                                                                          CIP

Printed in the United States of America

First Edition

1 2 3 4 5 6 7 8 9 10

BOOK DESIGN BY ANN GOLD

We lovingly dedicate
Gifts of Time
to
"The Children"

PREFACE

Gifts of Time is a true story. All the case histories are based on fact. But to protect the privacy of the pediatric patients and their families, we have altered many of their names, genders, and sometimes, social backgrounds. In some instances, two or more case histories have been blended.

We wrote this book for many reasons. The major one is to offer hope to the parents and families of very sick children. Such parents and families must find a way to access a medical system that all too often locks them out. We want them to know that there is never a good reason to surrender hope for any child.

ACKNOWLEDGMENTS

Having worked closely together for a year and a half, we find ourselves indebted to many friends, patients, and peers for their help and insights concerning this book.

Special thanks go to Peter B. Dunne, M.D.; Margarita Gonzalez; Margaret Masters, M.S., P.T.; Scott Pieper; Cameron K. Tebbi, M.D.; Ann Urbanski, and the dedicated staff of the Tampa/Hillsborough County Public Library. Thanks also to those who graciously answered every question—some more than once—and permitted us to use their actual names, including Rick Abbott, M.D.; Jeffrey Allen, M.D.; JoAnn Baldwin; Murray Canter, M.D.; Natalie Cutrone; Miriam Lubling; Joseph Ransohoff, M.D.; Rochelle Sedita; Tania Shiminski-Maher, R.N., M.S.; Jane Thurston; Julian Thurston; and Jeffrey Wisoff, M.D.

There are no words adequate enough to thank a most special group of people: the parents of the children represented in this book. They willingly shared their stories, their tears and despair, and their joys, in order to help those parents who would walk in their shoes.

Our most grateful thanks to our agents, Herb and Nancy

ACKNOWLEDGMENTS

Katz, who created the concept of this book, brought us together, and encouraged us throughout the research and writing.

We express gratitude to our editor, Adrian Zackheim,
whose sensitive responses to our manuscript were enormously
helpful.

A major thank-you also to our respective spouses, Hinks
and Kathy, for all their support and patience during the writing
of this book, especially the late-night telephone sessions. And
thanks too to our combined ten kids—The Shimberg Bunch:
Kasey, Scott, Betsy, Andy (and his bride, Cathy) and Michael; and the Epstein offspring: Samara, Ilana, Jason, Joseph,
and Benjamin. You guys kept us humble.

And very special thanks to Jean Arbeiter, friend and coun-
selor, whose invaluable suggestions are reflected throughout
the book.

GIFTS OF TIME

CHAPTER 1

There had been Dagners in Ashley, Mississippi, since before the Civil War. In what safer place could you bring up a child, Ina Bea and Clayton Dagner thought, than a small town where your family had lived for generations?

But Ashley, for all its lush Delta beauty, would fail young Kevin Dagner in a terrible way. He would nearly die because his town had no easy access to a major medical center, no specialist able to tell his parents what his mysterious symptoms might imply—or what should be done next. In fact, Kevin's story is typical of the way a sick child and his parents can become overwhelmed by terror simply because they don't know where to turn to get the help they need.

Until he was ten years old, Kevin had no story worth telling, not from a medical point of view, anyway. His life consisted of a succession of happy years, the kind that generally go unnoticed except by friends, teachers, and relatives. For Kevin's parents, Ina Bea and Clayton Dagner, these quiet years were a miracle.

Before Kevin's birth, they had despaired of ever having a

child. Ina Bea had experienced three miscarriages, and she was wary of Dr. Paterson's advice that she should "keep on trying." She didn't think she could endure one more loss, but Paterson had brought both Ina Bea and her husband into the world, and she had absolute faith in him. As it turned out, she was glad she took his advice.

Kevin grew from a lusty infant into a healthy, husky young boy, big-boned and tall, like his father. At ten, he looked more like a twelve-year-old. His height and strength gave him athletic prowess, but Kevin's popularity wasn't based on that alone. He was the kind of kid other kids took to, easygoing and amiable, yet totally true to his word. One of his teachers called him "the sunshine boy" because of his ready smile and helpful attitude. On Saturdays, Kevin assisted Clay in the family hardware store. The Dagners were proud of him.

Ina Bea couldn't recall when she first noticed a physical change in her son. In the beginning, it was almost imperceptible—a slight hesitation in his walk, a need to hold on tightly to the banister when he went up the stairs. What bothered her most was her feeling that he was holding something back, but she decided not to pry. The mother of an only child can become overprotective, and she had long ago vowed not to subject Kevin to her own anxieties. She encouraged his aggressiveness on the soccer team, where he played goalie, though she dreaded his getting injured. She smiled as he and Clay left for early-morning hunting trips, though she couldn't stop herself from imagining all the dangers lurking in the nearby hills.

But now she didn't think she was imagining anything. She managed to keep silent for weeks until Kevin finally confided in her. He was feeling "funny," he said. His feet didn't work right anymore. What was particularly disturbing was the way the clumsiness was affecting his soccer game. It threw off his timing, and he could no longer kick the ball with his usual precision. His legs were acting like "a dopey pair of marionettes," with Kevin no longer pulling the strings. The coach was beginning to notice his problems, and so were his teammates. Kevin feared that he was letting them all down.

Clay, who took a matter-of-fact approach to everything, wondered if Kevin was undergoing some kind of growth spurt and could benefit from a different type of shoes, ones that would give him better support. Even after such shoes were purchased, and Kevin had worn them for a day or so, no change for the better was noticeable. Instead, Kevin struck Ina Bea as looking even more fatigued, his ready smile absent. She made an appointment with Dr. Paterson.

Dr. Paterson thought Kevin's problems could be caused by a virus, even though he had no fever. He speculated that an earlier fever could have gone unnoticed and that Kevin was suffering from the residue of the viral attack. He advised Ina Bea to keep Kevin at home for a few days, and in bed if possible, where he could build up his strength so that his body could recover.

Although Dr. Paterson spoke with his usual fatherly certainty, Ina Bea was uneasy. Somehow she had expected a more specific diagnosis, but felt she had no choice except to follow his advice. She called the nursery school where she taught, and advised the director that she would be at home for a week. Although Kevin was capable of staying alone, something told her it would be best to be with him.

Her premonition proved to be accurate. During that week, the headaches began. They came on just after Kevin awakened, but seemed to lessen as the day wore on. At their worst, they produced severe pain, and sometimes they made him vomit, just after he got out of bed.

And he held his head at a slight tilt most of the time now.

She noticed, too, that his difficulty in keeping his balance was becoming more pronounced, and that there was an increased weakness in his right leg. She was very frightened.

Ina Bea kept Kevin home another week, but there was no lessening of his symptoms. In the morning, she would find Kevin fighting back tears as he struggled to brush his teeth. The sight of her child in serious pain was tearing her apart. She insisted on making another trip to Dr. Paterson's office, this time with Clay in attendance.

Dr. Paterson revised his diagnosis when Ina Bea described the headaches and the vomiting. Kevin was probably suffering from migraines, he said. The boy was at the age when excruciating headaches of this sort often set in, particularly if they ran in families.

Clay remembered at that point that his grandfather had had migraines, and the doctor nodded knowingly, glad to have his thinking corroborated. Fortunately, he commented, there was medication available to control the pain, if Kevin took it when the headache first came on and tried to be more relaxed about things. Those soccer games, for example. He knew Kevin was proud to be goalie, but he had to learn to be less tense.

Clayton seemed reassured by the doctor's words, but for Ina Bea, the pieces didn't fit together. As the weeks went on, she found she was confiding in Clay less and less. Their dinner hour, once the time for a spirited interchange about the day's events, began to lag. Kevin ate little, reluctantly admitting that he was having difficulty getting the food down. He showed no interest even in his favorite dishes, excused himself from table early, and went to his room. In the morning, the headache reappeared. Clay insisted, though, that Ina Bea wasn't giving the medication enough time to work.

Gradually, Ina Bea realized that she couldn't trust Clay's

judgment, and for the first time in their relationship, she felt totally alone. Paterson's "just wait it out" advice was no comfort either.

One day the soccer coach brought Kevin home from practice because the boy was experiencing pain so severe that he could not walk.

Early the following morning, the Dagners were awakened by the sound of howls, like those of an animal being attacked. The noises, barely recognizable as human, came from the direction of Kevin's room.

When they pushed the door open, it was difficult to absorb what they saw. Kevin was on his knees in the middle of the bed, his face and pajamas covered with blood, his eyes closed. He rocked back and forth screaming, and as he screamed, he hacked at his left ear with his grandfather's hunting knife, a treasured possession usually kept on the night table.

Clay ordered Ina Bea to call the ambulance corps as he raced over to his son and wrested the knife out of his hand. As he did so, Kevin seemed to wake up. Clay picked up the boy's underpants from the floor and pressed the cotton fabric hard against the boy's ear. The material was quickly soaked with blood. Ina Bea found a bath towel, which they wrapped tightly around Kevin's head.

A few minutes later, they were in an ambulance on their way to the community hospital. Ina Bea sat in the back, a volunteer paramedic looking on, while she cradled her son in her arms. The towel had been replaced by a pressure bandage, and Kevin had been quieted with a sedative.

Suddenly she felt her son's chunky hand reach out for hers. He wanted to tell her something, he whispered. He'd had a bad dream, in which he was being chased by a tree. It was huge, a monster with a gnarled trunk and twisted branches. The tree caught up with Kevin, and its branches fastened on to his ear like a vise. The pain was searing. He had to fight off those branches.

In the emergency room, Dr. Paterson, who had been summoned from his bed, stitched up the wounds adeptly. Kevin's extreme behavior was unusual, he said, but migraines could sometimes drive patients to self-mutilation. He had to be frank, he went on, choosing his words carefully. He wondered if Kevin might be experiencing an emotional problem, and if a "mental health professional" might be of some assistance. Beyond that, he confessed, he could think of nothing to do.

At these words, Clay Dagner exploded. "You've known Kevin his whole life, Doctor. And he's as well balanced today as he ever was. We're not taking this child to a psychiatrist." Dr. Paterson shrugged, as if to say, "It's up to you."

The Dagners had no idea of where to turn next. All their lives they had trusted Dr. Paterson implicitly. He was their doctor, the person with all the answers. Now he had failed them. They didn't know any other physicians, nor did they know what type of specialist they needed. All of a sudden, Ashley, which had seemed like such a secure place to live, was secure no longer. Instead, it had become ominous in its isolation and limited knowledge.

After Kevin's release from the hospital the following day, the Dagners found themselves staring uneasily at each other in their living room. Kevin remained quiet, under sedation in his room. They didn't want to think about what tomorrow would be like. Their lives were no longer within their control. They were being controlled instead by an all-pervasive sense of horror.

Toward evening, Clay struggled to find something to think about besides his fear. Finally, he decided to go downstairs to his workroom, to clean it. That was just the kind of mindless activity he needed.

He directed all his energy toward tossing piles of old newspapers and magazines into a trash can. As he was picking up a stack of *Reader's Digests*, the cover of one yellowed issue caught his eye. Picking it up, he grew curious about an article called, "The Transformation of Aaron Alligator," which contained an illustration of a small boy lying helplessly in a hospital bed. "What happened to turn this bright laughing little boy into a stumbling, pain-racked waif?" the line above the title asked. It was the same question that Clay, unknown to Ina Bea, had been asking himself over the past months.

He began to read about a child who had been diagnosed as having a tumor on his spinal cord; the word "tumor" exploded off the page at Clay.

Reading further, he learned that the boy's tumor was considered to be inoperable until a neurosurgeon in Manhattan succeeded in removing it, using a technique he had recently invented. The surgeon's name was Fred Epstein, and he was at New York University Medical Center.

Clay ripped out the article, folded it carefully, and put it in his pocket. As he walked up the stairs, he felt his heart pounding wildly. "Don't use the phone," he called out to Ina Bea when he reached the landing. "I'm going to call New York."

CHAPTER 2

Not even the late-fall darkness can mask the bleakness of New York on one of those days when tension and sheer ugliness overwhelm the city's images of glamour and power. Although it was only three in the afternoon, the buildings of New York University Medical Center were already shrouded in gray.

Still, they maintained their authority. Sprawling down First Avenue, from Thirty-fourth to Twenty-fourth streets, the complex dominated the neighborhood, not by virtue of its architecture, which is decidedly nondescript, but because of its importance as one of the world's largest and best medical centers.

The street was crowded with people heading in and out of the center's doors. There were professionals and technicians in medical whites, young families with children in strollers, and the elderly, many of whom pushed walkers or were themselves being pushed along in wheelchairs. At curbside, a phalanx of taxis deposited passengers and picked up others.

JoAnn Baldwin watched as a stout, middle-aged man helped an elderly gentleman, perhaps his father, out of a car, then raced around to the back to take a pair of crutches out of the trunk. There's never an end to the "customers," she thought, never an end to the need for help. In all her years as Dr. Fred Epstein's office manager, JoAnn had not gotten used to it, particularly since their patients—she thought of the patients as being hers as well as Fred's—were young children with terrible illnesses. Yet she knew that she thrived, as her boss did, in an atmosphere of crisis combined with caring.

JoAnn walked along briskly, clutching her black cape tightly around her for protection against the East River winds. She was a strong, robust woman, no taller than five foot two, and the cape fell almost to her ankles. She stepped gingerly over newspapers and swirling debris, all the while aware of the cacophony of languages around her. Spanish, Yiddish, and Arabic were just a few she could identify.

A family of Jamaicans followed JoAnn as she ducked into the Howard A. Rusk Institute of Rehabilitation Medicine, where Fred Epstein's office was located. Inside, they milled around in the narrow, claustrophobic entryway, wondering what to do next. JoAnn regarded them sympathetically. The directory was not within easy sight, so it often fell to a guard to direct visitors and make sure that they didn't get lost. After pointing the Jamaicans toward the right elevator, the guard greeted JoAnn.

"Where's your doctor today? I haven't seen him."

"He had to go to a funeral," JoAnn replied.

"Oh."

There was no need to comment further. In spite of Fred's successes, not all of the children he operated on lived to grow up. There was no way for anyone who didn't work with Fred to know how much these endings tormented him. They tore him to pieces, because he became a part of the families he treated, visiting them at home, attending birthday parties and other celebrations, and making himself available by phone at any time.

"Why can't you just cut and go?" another surgeon once asked him. "You get too involved with your patients, Fred. It's not good."

"Not good for whom?" Fred had answered. "I *know* it's good for the parents. They tell me it is. You know, they become my patients, too. They carry an incredible burden. They need to know you really care, that it goes beyond what you do in the hospital. It's important for the family to feel that they can come in and talk whenever they need to. They have to be able to feel hope."

"That's just it," his colleague replied. "How can you offer hope when you know there isn't any?"

"You have to believe," Fred said. "Miracles do happen. I've seen them happen."

The thought of the funeral sent a sudden chill through JoAnn. Reflexively, she pulled her cape closer around her. A feeling of sadness overcame her, and she had to fight back tears. Get yourself together, girl, she thought, or get out of this kind of work.

But difficult as days like today were, JoAnn couldn't imagine working anyplace else. For the past nine years, she had been the ringmaster and chief juggler of Fred Epstein's three-ring medical circus, overseeing a staff of two office assistants, and serving as mother hen to a parade of interns and residents. The practice covered the care of children with brainstem tumors and spinal cord tumors, and with other central nervous system disorders, such as hydrocephalus and spina bifida.

It was JoAnn who fielded the continuous phone calls from physicians and frantic parents, putting first one, then another person on hold while she tossed questions to Fred or his partners, Jeff Wisoff and Rick Abbott. She cataloged the twenty or more sets of diagnostic films that came in weekly from physicians around the world, wanting Fred's opinion of their patients' chances. Was an operation advisable, or was it not? They all needed answers—and quickly.

JoAnn kept track of Fred's appointments, typed his papers, ordered his lunch, and reminded him about family birthdays and anniversaries. For Fred's intense concentration on his patients was matched by pure absentmindedness when it came to the details of everyday life, much to the distress of Kathy, his wife of twenty-seven years.

A job description for JoAnn's particular position would have to include the word "soldier" because Fred ran a medical crusade, not just an office. "Kids aren't meant to be sick," he would say emphatically. "They're certainly not meant to die." He was prepared to pull out every stop to hold death at bay. "With children," he often reminded the residents who congregated in his office, "the mandate is different than with adults. You give an adult four to five extra years, and he can settle his affairs. The mandate with a kid is to be aggressive, so he can live. What's four to five years to a child?"

Everyone who worked with Fred absorbed his commitment to saving every child—no matter how much extra time and effort he and his staff had to give. That commitment entailed putting in long hours, or coming in at strange times of day as well as being there for parents who had traveled from far away and were tired, frightened, and confused. It meant handing them a cup of coffee, offering a moment's comfort, and negotiating with the hospital bureaucracy to make their lives simpler. There were many rewards, like seeing a child who had arrived at the center sobbing in agony, return one day for a checkup with a steadier walk and a ready smile. Another reward was feeling good when you went home at night.

It occurred to JoAnn that she even loved the craziness of

the place, the ringing phones, the last-minute schedule changes, and the odd turns. Like today, for example, when she had to search for a file that turned out to be buried in the storage section of an adjacent building. Fred had suddenly thought that it might be related to a case he was working on currently, but as usual he wasn't quite sure where the file might be or exactly when he had operated. And, as usual, it fell to JoAnn to straighten things out.

As she pushed the elevator button, file in hand, JoAnn heard familiar footsteps coming up behind her. She turned to see Fred Epstein, director of pediatric neurosurgery, loping down the hall in the half-awkward, half-graceful fashion that was his normal gait. Tanned and trim, and standing more than six feet tall, he looked like a man more at home on a tennis court or in a sailboat than in an operating room, peering through a microscope and probing a child's delicate brain.

His honey-blond hair was beginning to thin somewhat and show some gray around the temples, but at fifty-three, he maintained an astonishingly boyish appearance. Perhaps it was his open face and easy manner, a manner that left him only under the most adverse circumstances. In fact, JoAnn knew, Fred's engaging grin, which Kathy, his wife, called his "Blackburn smile," could hide a variety of feelings, particularly on a day like this one. (Joseph Blackburn was an eighteenth-century artist who painted more than a hundred subjects with the corners of their mouths turned up, just like Fred's.)

"How did it go?" JoAnn asked as they stepped into the elevator. The funeral had been for Davy Feldman, a twelve-year-old Fred had first operated on two years ago. Since then there had been one more operation on Davy, then the sad realization that nothing further could be done.

"Max and Ruth Feldman asked me to sit with them," Fred replied softly. "They said I was part of the family."

A muscle in his cheek twitched involuntarily. JoAnn knew he had revealed as much as he could. At times like these, Fred struggled to work through his emotions, sharing them with no one, not even Kathy, whom he called his best friend. Kathy—and the staff—knew when to step back and let him be.

JoAnn had spoken with Ruth Feldman just a week or so before Davy's death. "Fred's always been there for us," Ruth said, "for Davy, too. A lot of doctors would have taken a walk when things got bad."

But this doctor, JoAnn thought, hadn't taken a walk, and the strain showed in his bent shoulders and uncharacteristically subdued manner.

Getting off the elevator on the fifth floor, Fred and JoAnn walked toward Fred's office. On their way, they had to pass through the rehabilitation unit, which was filled with disabled youngsters, seated in Lilliputian wheelchairs or struggling to master a variety of equipment. Instead of natural giggles and laughter, these children emitted subdued groans and soft cries.

A toddler, balanced precariously on braces, lunged toward a physical therapist, who encouraged him with outstretched arms.

"Come to me, Jesse. You can do it," she coaxed.

Another therapist worked on the stubborn spastic muscles of an older child, who lay on a small gurney, her eyes staring listlessly into space. A few feet away, a little girl with twisted feet rode laboriously back and forth on a tricycle with super-large pedals.

JoAnn knew that many visitors to Fred's office found the rehabilitation unit unnerving. They would look straight ahead to avoid the struggling bodies, and thus missed the fierce looks of determination on the small, sweat-covered faces. But both Fred and JoAnn took strange comfort from the children's confirmation of that mysterious will to live.

Fred smiled at the girl on the tricycle. "Hey, young lady. You're looking good today." He reached down and patted her on the shoulder. The gesture was a familiar one, JoAnn thought, for Fred was a toucher. She had often seen him hug not only his young patients, but their parents as well. Physical contact came naturally to him. It broke down the barriers between the medical and the human, between the competent caregiver and the anxious recipient of care. "We're all in this together," was Fred's attitude, and it showed.

The girl on the tricycle grinned back at Fred, and for a moment his mood seemed to elevate. But by the time he and JoAnn arrived at his office, he had become somber again.

Suite 518 was in its usual state of seeming chaos. Each of the six phones was ringing, and JoAnn's two co-workers, Rochelle Sedita and Natalie Cutrone, were doing their best to answer the callers' questions. The computer screen on JoAnn's desk flashed some sort of message, which no one had time to respond to. Several drawers in the massive bank of file cabinets were open, and mounds of files lay on the floor, waiting to be put away. In a corner, Tania Shiminski-Maher, Fred's nurse-practitioner, leaned against the copying machine, compiling a list of patients for him to see when he made rounds.

Everywhere there was evidence of food deliveries—past and present—on desks and chairs and cabinets. A pizza box, with half a pizza in it, empty Chinese food containers, unopened soda cans, and a few bags of potato chips. The office seemed to be fueled on order-ups and carry-outs. Fred and the staff munched constantly, not only because they were too busy to go out, but also to break the tension. Food was so reassuring in the midst of illness and uncertainty.

Normally, the staff would have greeted Fred jovially or with the steady banter that characterized their relationship. But today there had been a funeral. Everyone quieted down when he walked in, and even the relentless telephones seemed to fall silent momentarily.

It was 3:30, but JoAnn was aware that Fred had almost a full day's work ahead of him. Time to get down to business, she thought. Don't give him too much of a chance to think.

She handed him a pile of pink oversized CALL BACK slips. "They all need to hear from you right away, especially Dr. Brown. He wants to know when we're going to schedule his patient. And Kathy called to remind you about the lecture series tonight at the Metropolitan Museum of Art."

Fred stuffed the slips in the pocket of his navy blue suit. "Anything else?" he asked.

"Yes, remember the Dagners, the family referred to you by Dr. Sparks at that large medical center in Mississippi? I think you're the one who sent them to Sparks originally. Anyway, they'll be here soon."

Fred nodded, running over the details of the Dagner case in his mind. His face took on a concerned expression. JoAnn knew how much he hated a story of delayed diagnosis like Kevin's, with its loss of precious time and infliction of additional pain. Tania, who had admitted Kevin late last night, told JoAnn that she had rarely seen a child in so much pain. The resources of major medical centers should be readily available to all parents, Fred thought. Too many families got lost in the cracks, unable to get the help they needed. At least this family had been fortunate enough to connect with him.

JoAnn, too, felt a twinge of emotion thinking of the Dagners. Just like her boss, she was always affected when a new case began. Her heart would reach out to the family, even before she met them. She could sense the terror in their voices as they spoke to her on the phone. They had been told their child would die unless they could get to Fred Epstein or one of the few other pediatric neurosurgeons in the country who attempted the risky surgery he did.

They would arrive carrying this burden of terror with them, looking for someplace to diminish it, to lay it down. That place was Fred's office. Here he would dissect the terror, put it under a microscope, and help them to carry it by taking some of it on himself. Here, in this office, he would start a relationship that made each set of parents believe his feeling for them was unique. The truth was, he cared about all of them equally, but his involvement in each case was so intense that it seemed to shut out all others. No wonder he was absentminded about getting to dinner parties, or even just plain dinner.

"Don't forget to call Kathy," JoAnn reminded Fred. If the Dagners were late, he might well miss the lecture at the Metropolitan, leaving Kathy to go alone. Some advance notice would be nice, but she didn't always get it.

"Your wife is a saint to put up with you," JoAnn had commented on more than one occasion.

"She can't be a saint; we're Jewish," Fred would shoot back. But JoAnn knew that he agreed with her assessment of Kathy.

Fred headed toward his office and motioned to Tania Shiminski-Maher to come along.

The commodious office was empty. Usually there was some sort of conference going on, groups of residents looking at magnetic resonance imaging films, commonly called MRIs, or Fred's associates would be discussing a procedure. It could get pretty crowded at times, with staff members walking in and out at will, but Fred was able to concentrate and go on with his work. In fact, a hubbub in the background seemed to have a salutary effect on him.

Now, it seemed to Tania, the silence was making Fred uneasy. He glanced out the grime-streaked window at the city's heliport down below and watched the lights of a copter maneuvering in for a landing. Then, settling himself in a leather chair, he pushed aside the files on his disorderly desk, making room for the pile of pink slips. He leaned back, sprawling his long legs under the desk and kicking aside a pair of green operating room clogs that had nested there.

Tania leaned forward in her chair, pushing her glasses up on her nose. She was a pleasant-looking young woman whose subdued manner belied her extreme intelligence and her ability to help families in crisis. It was Tania's job to explain to parents in understandable language what was happening to their children, to stay with them during the operation, and to work with them afterward in adjusting to rehabilitation and to an illness that might recur. Like Fred, Tania had to be able to go deep into a family's collective psyche to discover the strengths that would allow them to cope or identify problems that might prevent their coping.

Tania handed Fred the list of patients he had to see on rounds, with their room numbers clearly marked. Several years ago, Fred, in his sometimes distracted manner, had wandered into the wrong patient's room and proceeded to discuss someone else's operation. After that episode, Tania had taken on the chore of pointing him in the proper direction.

"I'm afraid there's bad news," she said as Fred looked over the list. "Sarah Glazer has been readmitted. And the scan on Luis Olmedo isn't good."

She produced a file containing MRI films with the name "Olmedo" in the upper right-hand corner. Jeff Wisoff, Fred's associate, had spent a considerable amount of time looking at the films, Tania reported. They showed that the seven-year-old boy's spinal cord tumor, a malignant astrocytoma that Fred had operated on three years ago, had begun to grow again. Another operation would be necessary. Jeff was setting up a conference right now with Luis's mother on Nine East, the pediatric floor, where twenty beds were reserved for neurosurgery and oncology patients.

Fred took the file somewhat reluctantly, Tania thought. She knew he dreaded having to look at the bad news, particularly when he had hoped against hope there would be no recurrence of the tumor. The file's contents, the topping to a dismal day, were sure to produce a new wave of negative emotions.

It didn't matter how many of his patients were doing well. Fred agonized over those who weren't. He didn't take the risks he took, remove the tumors that others considered unremovable, so that children could continue to suffer. Still, at bottom he was realistic. Recurrence was always a possibility, and so was death. It was the quality of the time in between that was important, he said. And for many, that quality time could stretch out into a normal life span. The shuffle of the cards was not totally unpredictable—benign tumors responded far better to treatment than did malignant ones—but it was a shuffle nonetheless.

Tania glanced at a plaque on the wall that read: THE BRAINSTEM IS A HIGHLY OVERRATED ORGAN. It had been given to Fred as a tongue-in-cheek tribute by his colleague Michael Edwards in San Francisco. In the early eighties, Fred had appeared there as a visiting professor, presenting a lecture describing which brainstem tumors could and could not be operated on. Prior to then, the brainstem had been considered an "inoperable" area. The plaque attested to the fact that the scalpel—in the form of its successors, high-tech instruments—could now traverse the tiny organ with something resembling impunity.

A few years later, Fred entered forbidden territory again, becoming the first neurosurgeon to remove an astrocytoma that ran the length of a child's spinal cord. He had since performed the delicate operation on seventy children, of whom Luis Olmedo was one.

But for all of Fred's expertise, the brainstem and the spinal cord remained tough challenges for a surgeon, and a tumor could fight back. When one did, it took the wind out of Fred. But only temporarily. Tania knew that soon he would be fighting, too, employing all of his surgical skills, and the skills of his colleagues, the oncologists and radiation therapists, to save Luis.

Right now, though, he needed some bolstering himself. Under a pile of papers on Fred's desk, Tania saw the bulge of a familiar file folder. In this folder, JoAnn shoved the letters and photographs that arrived regularly from grateful parents, many of them writing more than once. It wasn't unusual for Fred to keep up a steady correspondence with parents, even those he no longer saw on yearly checkup visits. But the letters in this file were something special. They were all upbeat, his reward for a job well done. Tania guessed the file was on Fred's desk now because JoAnn had made some recent additions.

She pulled out the folder and opened it. On top there was a color snapshot of a muscular teenager in a baseball uniform. The attached letter read, "As you can see, Bart is doing beautifully. It's been five years, and there's no sign of recurrence, thank God. The operation seems like a bad dream, almost, but it's not forgotten. Bart's captain of the junior varsity team now. We can never thank you enough."

Tania looked at the picture with pleasure. Except for the scar under the rear hairline, hidden in the photograph by a baseball cap, no one who met the boy would have guessed he had once been so seriously ill.

She flipped through the pile of letters and postcards. "Greeting from Valley Forge," said one. Others were postmarked

Coeur d'Alene, Idaho, and Piraeus, Greece. The little Greek girl stared at the camera with huge brown eyes and a shy smile. On the back, her mother had written, "For Dr. Fred, the man who gave our daughter back her life." A letter from Bahia, Brazil, was written on thin notebook paper, the printing shaky. "The language is an immense barrier, but I have for you an immense affection as only a mother can have." She had obtained the services of a translator, the woman went on to say, to make certain she was expressing her feelings correctly.

Tania straightened up the letters, so that they no longer stuck out of the folder in a haphazard fashion. Fred had turned his back to her and was starting to insert the Olmedo films into the viewer.

"Why don't you look at these letters first?" Tania asked. "I think you have some time before the Dagners come." She handed him the file. Then she strode quickly toward the door and exited, her neatly polished brown loafers carrying her along soundlessly.

CHAPTER 3

FRED

I pushed the file aside. All the accolades in the world don't mean a thing when you've just come from a patient's funeral.

Not when you've had to sit there and listen as a father delivers the eulogy for his twelve-year-old son. Max Feldman actually thanked me for my "unshakable belief that nearly anything was possible, that Davy might live a full life."

I felt absolutely rotten. How much Davy wanted to live, I well knew. He loved life so much that he couldn't wait to get out of bed in the morning; that is, until he could no longer get out of bed at all, but lay there, his face so bloated from steroids that the features were unrecognizable.

"How come you sawed my brain out?" he asked me once.

I explained a little bit at a time, the way you have to with children and adolescents. Davy learned that he had a brain tumor, a mixed astrocytoma ependymoma. While most tumors of this type are slow-growing and benign, the indications were that Davy's would be different. That was why I acted quickly and "sawed" away at his brain.

I remembered my first meeting with Max and Ruth Feldman as vividly as if it had been this morning. Ruth, short and buxom, with strong coloring, chattered away to hide nervousness, twisting her leather gloves in her hands.

"Dr. Epstein. We've heard so much about you from our friend Diane Lewis. Do you remember her?" I shook my head. "Well, she came here once with her boy. I forget his name. Max, what was Diane Lewis's younger boy's name?"

Max shrugged without pausing to think. He was a slightly paunchy, full-faced man who seemed ten to fifteen years his wife's senior. He sat patiently on my maroon leather couch, waiting for Ruth to pause for breath. When she did, he patted her arm gently, then turned to me.

"Well, Dr. Epstein, you've seen Davy's tests. What are his chances?"

I never hedge. Parents need to know that they can trust me to be frank, because we'll be working together for a long time.

"It's a tumor and a bad one," I said honestly. "It's in the brainstem, which makes it very serious." Ruth gasped, but I went on. "Davy needs surgery, and quickly. I'll make arrangements to operate on Friday."

Ruth Feldman was strangely quiet. Max spoke up. "Can you get it all?"

"No, but I can remove enough to be hopeful it won't come back." In a gentle tone, I went on to describe the possible side effects of the surgery I was proposing. "Davy might have trouble breathing or swallowing. There could be body paralysis. Facial paralysis, too. He might even die."

I held nothing back. I knew I was overloading them, that they were hearing my words but not processing them all.

Tonight the reality would begin to seep in, and in the days ahead, more and more until it became the dominant theme of their lives.

"Go home and rest now," I told the Feldmans at last. "My door is always open. Write down any questions you can think of. Call me if you need to. My number's in the phone book."

That information shocked Ruth out of her silence. "You have a listed number?" I nodded. "I can't believe that," she said. "A doctor with a listed home phone." She nudged her husband. "Max, can you believe that?" Max shook his head.

I had to smile at the memory. Ruth always spoke her mind, even right from the beginning. And she continued to do so, until the end, an end that was far worse than I could have prepared her for.

As Davy's illness progressed, Ruth and I developed a real rapport. I became accustomed to her nervous chatter, learning that it masked both strength and a fierce love for her son.

Ruth was tough, but she was realistic as well. When Davy turned twelve, she stopped by my office. "Fred, we've got to talk about his bar mitzvah," she said.

"Davy's just twelve, Ruth. Boys become bar mitzvah at thirteen."

"Will he be here then?" she asked simply.

I looked back at her and found myself caught by her gaze. "I hope so, Ruth," I said, respecting her too much to lie, "but I honestly don't know. Davy's not responding as well as I'd hoped to any of the drugs."

"Those drugs are affecting his memory," she said wearily. "He can't remember what he had to eat yesterday. It's harder for him to walk, too, and even to swallow. He chokes on his own saliva."

"What are you thinking?" I asked.

"I want him to have his bar mitzvah this year, along with

his brother Jonathan, who's a year older. Jonathan can help hold Davy when he loses his balance and read both parts from the Torah, if he has to. I want it for Davy, before it's too late. And I want you to come, Fred, to read a blessing." She blurted it out in one sentence, as though she feared I might interrupt if she paused.

I smiled. "That's great. Sure, I'd be honored to take part. I'm a regular at Saturday morning synagogue services during the summer on Fire Island. My Hebrew's pretty good. I'll look forward to it."

And go I did, thrilled to witness not only an ancient coming-of-age ceremony for two boys, but also the magical power of hope and love. Davy Feldman, supported by Jonathan, stood swaying slightly but proudly before the congregation, his tiny bald head covered by a blue velvet yarmulke. Breaking into a lopsided grin that seemed to envelop his wizened face, Davy recited as much of the traditional prayers as he could. Although the words were somewhat slurred, due to his poor muscle coordination, I thought they were moving and sweet.

"It was the most wonderful bar mitzvah I've ever attended," I told Ruth afterward at the reception in the synagogue's social hall, "including my own."

It had been special. But then Davy was a special kid. "They're all special," I announced now to the empty room. But why, I wondered, do the kids who die haunt my memory so? Even as I asked, I knew the answer. Watching a tumor ravage a child is like watching all the beauty of creation in reverse, like a black mass of some sort. It wasn't meant to be that way. Children weren't meant to die; yet in my twenty-two years as a neurosurgeon, I've certainly observed that they do.

I don't accept it, though, until I've tried everything, gone the whole distance. I take on cases that other neurosurgeons shy away from, because I don't believe in the "inevitable," at least not until I've made it stand up and strike me in the face.

Then it knocks me out.

Well, nobody forced you into this specialty, I said to myself. You could have been a general practitioner or a pediatrician. It was you who always wanted to go to the edge, who needed to be where it's hot.

Maybe I get that need from my psychiatrist father, who took risks, too, sometimes administering insulin shock therapy to catatonic patients more frequently than was the norm. One patient failed to respond after ten treatments; yet Dad did it again, after the rest of the staff had closed the book. I was on summer break from college then, and I served as an aide at the private mental hospital my father owned.

"This time may be different," he told me. "Maybe this treatment is the one that will work. You can't always believe what everybody tells you. You have to go all the way." And the patient did respond, went on to get well, but my father could just as easily have fallen on his face. Just as I had with Davy Feldman.

And now, Luis Olmedo? Looking at the MRI films, I could see that the news was indeed bad. Damn! I slammed the pictures down on my desk. I could never get used to how angry these tumors made me. I wanted to annihilate each evil cell, the classical doctor-as-God complex. I didn't need my father to tell me that, or to point out that it was unhealthy. Still, I couldn't shake off the anger.

I had removed about 80 percent of Luis's malignant astrocytoma. It was impossible to remove any more because the tumor had become intermeshed with the spinal cord's delicate nerve network. What remained of the tumor was treated with radiation and chemotherapy and, for the past three years, Luis had been, as we say, "clean."

I knew that Jeff Wisoff, my brilliant associate, would set up a conference for me with Carmen Olmedo, Luis's mother, as tactfully as possible. But I wasn't looking forward to talking with her at that meeting.

Since the Olmedos came from Ecuador and spoke no English, it was necessary to communicate through an interpreter. That created a barrier between us, a barrier reinforced by the formality of Carmen's proud Indian manner. I always had the feeling that she was keeping something from me, something more than fear, which I think she disdained to reveal to an outsider.

Luis had become my patient in a way that can only be called miraculous. One day, Carmen, carrying the boy in her arms, found her way to a World Health Organization clinic in Guayaquil that happened to be run by one of my former residents.

I received the call at home.

"Hello, Fred, this is Don Brickelmeyer. I think we've got a four-year-old kid with a spinal cord tumor here."

The symptoms had come on quickly, Brickelmeyer explained, severe pain along the spinal axis, difficulty in walking, a burning sensation in the fingers and toes, and an impaired sense of touch. Now Luis could barely move.

"I have a feeling we're getting far along here," Brickelmeyer commented.

He meant that he feared the tumor was extensive and malignant.

"Let me take a look at the boy," I said.

"Fred, I'm in the slums of Guayaquil," he replied.

I told Brickelmeyer that I'd have JoAnn call him back and arrange for a flight. He'd have to help the Olmedos with passports and visa arrangements. But the tickets, the surgery, and the hospitalization would be on me and NYU, helped by special funding that has been developed over the years for families who can't afford the costs.

Waiving my fee is my way of paying back the good fortunes of my life, maybe even a way to keep the evil eye far from my own five children. I never look at a child like Luis, in drugged sleep on the operating table, without thinking it could just as well have been one of mine lying there. In fact, being in this business has made me pretty much of a worrier. Whenever my eighteen-year-old, Ilana, has a migraine, I'm a wreck. Every time six-year-old Joey has an asthma attack, my heart is in my mouth.

"Calm down, Doctor," Kathy has pleaded with me many times.

There was a knock at the door.

"The Dagners are here," JoAnn announced.

Ina Bea and Clay Dagner looked weary and bewildered, yet relieved finally to make contact with me. They were a Jack Sprat couple, Clay's tall and muscular physique contrasting with his wife's plump softness and short stature. Years of living together, no doubt, had given them the same open expression, the same straightforward look I had seen on their son Kevin when I examined him early this morning before going to Davy Feldman's funeral.

"What a beautiful quilt," Ina Bea remarked in a soft southern voice as she and Clay sat down on the leather sofa. Above the sofa, and occupying one entire wall, hung a nineteenth-century American quilt, part of a collection Kathy and I have been building for years.

"Thank you," I said, pulling up a chair so that I could sit opposite them. I don't like putting a desk between me and parents, preferring to be where I can make eye contact and touch them in a reassuring way, if need be. At this first moment, I start to build the bond that will have to support us all through difficult times.

Clay Dagner took the *Reader's Digest* article out of his pocket and smoothed it on his knee. Obviously, he had carried it as a talisman ever since the day he'd called me in terror two weeks ago. I'd referred the Dagners to Dr. Harold Sparks, a neurologist who practiced about two hours from their home. He had examined Kevin and then ordered a magnetic resonance imaging scan.

The MRI scanner is a piece of equipment shaped like a tunnel. The patient lies on a table that slides into the tunnel, where his head is subjected to a very strong magnetic field and to radio-frequency energy. These forces produce a series of magnetic absorption images, which are later transferred to film.

Because the MRI can "see through" bone, which can obstruct other types of scanner images, it provides a clear picture of the brain, even distinguishing, for example, between white and gray matter. Since its introduction a decade ago, the MRI has made the diagnosis of brain tumors a great deal easier. The scan not only identifies whether or not there is a tumor, but accurately shows in most cases how far it has spread.

In Kevin's case, the news was not good. Dr. Sparks had found a glioma, one of the most common types of brain tumor. This one appeared to be an astrocytoma, a tumor arising from the astrocyte cells, which form part of the supportive tissue of the brain and are named for their starlike shape. The intracranial pressure caused by Kevin's growing tumor accounted for his poor coordination, headaches, and loss of appetite.

Clay Dagner cleared his throat, while Ina Bea clung to his

arm, too frightened to speak. I could see that he wanted to choose his words carefully.

"Dr. Sparks sent us here. He said that very few people would operate on a tumor like Kevin's. And I was thinking, well, wondering really . . ."

"Why other doctors won't?"

"Yes."

The reason, I explained to the Dagners, was the location of Kevin's tumor, in the brainstem. The tiny brainstem—only an inch to an inch and a half thick and actually an extension of the spinal cord—is the final common pathway to everything, controlling basic functions such as blood pressure, heartbeat, movement, and breathing. Operating in this area with conventional instruments was considered impossible because of the multiple vital functions that could be damaged.

At the word "breathing," I heard Ina Bea gasp, but I continued because I had to make her understand that surgery was the one way to save Kevin's life. Until recently, tumors like his had been treated only with radiation or chemotherapy; and even though patients might improve temporarily, they inevitably died within two years.

"How do you do it then?" Clay asked.

"It" meant the surgery, a word that I've found many parents hesitate to use.

A number of new advances made my work possible, I said. One was the laser, which, when focused at close range, is capable of immense heat and power. It destroys tumor cells by vaporizing them. Another tool was the one Clay had read about in the Reader's Digest article, the Cavitron Ultrasonic Surgical Aspirator (CUSA), a pencil-like instrument devised for brain surgery by researchers at New York University Medical Center and the Cavitron Corporation, now Valley Lab in Boulder, Colorado. The Cavitron tip vibrates at 23,000 times a second, virtually liquefying tumor tissue and then suctioning it out.

High-tech instruments like these allowed me to dissect a tumor without having to exert pressure on surrounding areas, such as the one that controlled breathing.

I didn't mention my other tools: sheer nerve, and the belief that their son could be saved.

I told the Dagners that I suspected that Kevin's tumor was not malignant. It appeared to be confined rather than diffuse or infiltrating; it was probably a low-grade tumor. Tumors are graded according to their malignancy and tendency to spread. Those that have not infiltrated are termed low-grade tumors; those that have infiltrated are called mid- and high-grade tumors.

I thought I could remove a good part of Kevin's tumor, I told his parents, demonstrating with my hands how the surrounding tissue would be pulled back and the tumor pulverized by instruments.

I didn't downplay the dangers—paralysis or some loss of motor function—but there was a good chance Kevin would return to his normal self. I've operated on over eighty brainstem tumors, and in cases like Kevin's, the results were usually good.

"Will he ever play soccer again?" Ina Bea spoke up.

"I hope so. Hey, I expect you to invite me to the first game when he does."

For the first time, Ina Bea's round face seemed to relax a little, and the slightest trace of a smile appeared. Clay still looked at me formally and sat with his back straight, as if he were sitting on a court bench.

I couldn't blame him for judging me. After all, he was deciding whether or not to let a perfect stranger open his son's head and dig deep inside it with instruments that must have sounded to him like pure science fiction.

Clay Dagner wet his lips. I expected him to ask for time to think it over, but instead he asked, "When will you do it?"

"Tomorrow."

He started slightly.

"It's not a medical emergency, but Kevin's in horrible pain. I think we can make him feel better. There's no reason to wait."

Clay nodded in agreement. "Do it," he whispered.

Ina Bea Dagner began to sob quietly, reaching into her handbag for a scrunched-up lace handkerchief that she had clearly given plenty of use.

I moved my chair closer and took her hand. "I want you to know, we're in this together. I'm available whenever you need me. And Tania will be with you every moment she can while the operation is going on."

Mrs. Dagner nodded and put down the handkerchief, and I could see determination growing in her clear gray eyes.

"Listen," I said, "I intend to take that tumor out. I will take it out, but I have to feel you're with me. We're a team."

"I'm with you, Doctor," Clay Dagner murmured.

Ina Bea looked at him.

"I think I want to go back upstairs with Kevin now," she said.

"That's a good idea," I replied.

"He's my only child," she stated simply.

She didn't have to add, "And I'm putting him in your hands." I knew all too well what it meant to carry the life of someone else's child. All too well how it felt to save such a child, or lose one, or perhaps even worse, to leave one totally paralyzed. I glanced up at the plaque on the wall, the one about the brainstem being an overrated organ. I can do it, I reminded myself. I've been there before. I can make Kevin Dagner well.

Clay Dagner helped his wife to her feet. "By the way," he said, as he opened the door, "one of the parents up there, a Rabbi Glazer, asked us to say Hi to you. He said he'll see you later, when you make rounds."

"Hi." For Rabbi Daniel Glazer, scholar and mystic, it was a simple message, perhaps the simplest I'd received from him in the eleven years of our relationship.

I'd operated on Rabbi Glazer's daughter Sarah when she was six months old, a healthy infant suddenly stricken with a massive seizure. She was on the operating table the morning after a New Jersey hospital rushed her to me.

When I opened up Sarah's tiny skull, I saw an enormous bifrontal tumor, filling a third of her cranium. I removed a small bit of the tumor for biopsy, but I knew damn well it was malignant and that the case was hopeless.

I answered the Glazers' frantic questions as honestly as I knew how. There was no way to remove all of the tumor, and an infant that young could not undergo radiation because of the brain damage it would cause. No matter what was done surgically, the tumor would recur in short order. "Take her home and love her a lot," I told Daniel and his wife, Lila. "She's got about six months, I think, maybe a little more."

Sarah proved me wrong. The malignant tumor started to shrink, and for the first few years of her life, Sarah developed fairly normally. "She could have passed for a well child," was how Lila put it.

There was no way to account for Sarah's survival, but mine wasn't the first medical prediction that proved to be incorrect. The fact is that no two cancers are really alike. Medical students always are surprised when I tell them that, but it's true. Even if two tumors are similar and the outcome fairly predictable, there's no accounting for the human factor, that unique spark known as the human spirit. "That's what keeps doctors humble," I've reminded my residents more than once. "You can never say 'I'm sure.' "

Sarah had plenty of spirit. She kept me humble for three years; then her luck ran out. The tumor began to grow again, but now she was old enough to fight back.

After a fall from a jungle gym, Sarah suffered a cerebral hemorrhage. A malignant tumor, with blood vessels buried deep within it, hemorrhages easily.

Lila was consumed with guilt. "I just turned my back for a minute, Fred," she told me. "Please, don't let this be the end."

I looked at the scans with a neurologist. "Why bother to operate?" he asked in a flat tone.

"Because I have to do what I can," I told him.

I knew I could remove the clot and give Sarah a few more years, and I was right. It was a hairy operation. Sarah lost ten units of blood. I wouldn't have operated if I hadn't thought I could give her a few good years. But I never expected her to survive as long as she had and to experience so many ups and downs. Since the removal of the clot, I'd performed four more craniotomies, operations in which the skull is opened, on Sarah.

With each operation and course of follow-up treatment, I became closer to the Glazers. Now I was a member of their extended family. As with the Feldmans, I visited often in their home, sharing celebrations and even just quiet times. This is the only way I've found to experience what the parents of a chronically ill child endure and to give them the support they need.

My son Jason is just a few years older than Sarah, so we

had something in common when we met, with one major exception—Jason would live to grow up. Sarah was not expected to. "I never buy her a new winter coat," Lila once told me. Still Sarah would survive that winter, and then the next one, and then . . .

But now it didn't look as if there would be another "then." In recent months, Sarah's condition had deteriorated markedly. And there was so much scarring around previous operative sites that another operation would probably be impossible.

Yet I found myself holding back from sharing that news with the Glazers. Why? I had always been completely frank with them. Could it be that I was as hooked into the continuation of the miracle as they were? Or was it my own ego, my need to be the worker of miracles, that kept me from facing the truth?

Perhaps it had to do with my relationship with Daniel. He'd become more like a brother than a friend. Like me, Daniel was a searcher, I in the medical realm and he in the spiritual. There isn't as much difference between the two as we often think, particularly when critically ill children link them together.

I'm constantly tormented by the question of why innocent children become so ill, and Daniel, unlike many parents who are understandably concerned only with their own child, was able to universalize the issue. For him, Sarah's illness had to have some sort of purpose; but if it did, it changed the entire nature of the loving God he worshiped. For years, he was unable to resolve the quandary.

We'd have discussion after discussion, Daniel's piercing black eyes fixed on mine, as we stood outside of Sarah's hospital room or walked around the backyard of the Glazers' small suburban home.

For Daniel, I knew, it was an article of faith that Sarah would continue to survive. Lila was more realistic, but then she was closer to the situation, being the major caregiver.

Whip-smart and filled with energy, Lila had abandoned a promising career on Wall Street to stay home with her daughter. "Sarah's become my work," she confided to me during one visit.

Lila's life was totally circumscribed by her daughter's laborious care, while Daniel continued with his duties at a nearby congregation and as a teacher at the seminary. He was home as often as possible, but still, the major burden fell on Lila. Tensions grew.

This situation is not uncommon when a family has a chronically ill child. Almost inevitably, the illness creates a strain between the parents and between the parents and the well siblings. I've seen many cases where one spouse simply leaves, unable to endure the strain. Usually it's the father who walks out—Tania calls this the "Y chromosome syndrome"—but I remember one case in which a spinal cord patient was brought to me by her father after her mother had left.

However, I didn't expect the Glazers to break up. They were too devoted to one another. But an hour of truth was approaching for them, and for me, too. I reached for Sarah's file, which was buried in the clutter on my desk. It was thick, and I became weary at the thought of reviewing it again when almost every word was emblazoned on my memory.

I decided to discuss Sarah's case with the tumor board, a group of oncologists and other specialists that meets regularly Wednesday mornings to review cases and offer advice. I could use the input, I thought. Or was I kidding myself? I could guess what my colleagues' opinions would be. Coward, I told myself, buying time so you don't have to face Daniel and Lila.

I don't want to go to Sarah Glazer's funeral, I thought. Oh God, I don't want to go.

JoAnn poked her head in the door. "Jeff called to say that Mrs. Olmedo will be waiting for you in the library at six-thirty. And you still have to make rounds. And Kathy called."

I took Luis Olmedo's films out of the viewer and headed for the door, totally focused on him and the other children who awaited me on Nine East. Then I stopped and picked up the telephone.

It was only two seconds before I heard Kathy's bubbling voice on the other end of the line. "Hi! It's me," I said. "What's up?"

CHAPTER 4

Nine East doesn't look like the modern children's units promoted in hospital brochures, brightly lit and equipped with cozy furniture, toys, and decorations. There are no gingerbread houses painted on the walls, no balloons sprouting from the nurses' station. Instead, Nine East is plain, no-nonsense "hospital issue": light walls, well-trod linoleum, and minimal furniture in the small rooms. There is a view of the East River, if one is fortunate enough to get the bed near the window, but most of the children are too sick to enjoy it. Their parents try to make the rooms as homelike as possible, putting up posters and photographs.

Sarah Glazer's wall was papered with computer printouts, the results of her efforts on the laptop computer she kept with her at all times now. "I wish I could go out tomorrow with Naomi," one read. "Look at the moon," commented another.

Only Daniel and Lila Glazer knew the effort it cost Sarah to type out those statements. Her ability to speak was gone now, beyond the aid of the speech therapists who had helped her for many years, and her energy was severely diminished. Yet she insisted on communicating, insisted on remaining human when so little of her humanity was left.

Daniel Glazer glanced at his wife, asleep in an armchair across the room. Armchair was a misnomer, Daniel thought, for the plastic-covered arms were too narrow to rest one's arms comfortably and the seat was so spare that an occupant could barely shift about. Over the years, these chairs had constituted a particular instrument of torture for Daniel, yet Lila had adapted to them.

With each admission, she brought along a woolen afghan for warmth and a large soft pillow for the chair. By sewing an elastic strap to the back of the pillow, she could slip it over the chair and rest her back and head fairly comfortably.

That wasn't all of Lila's "hospital equipment." In the suitcase she kept packed at all times, there were changes of clothing, books, puzzles, toilet articles, and plastic bags of knitting and needlework projects. She also brought along personal photos, which she arranged on Sarah's night table, and an album of baby pictures of both Sarah and her older sister, Naomi. When Daniel commented on Lila's need to make the place so comfortable, Lila replied simply, "Why not? I live on the ninth floor of University Hospital."

The words, so full of truth, filled him with dread, confirming the implacability of Sarah's illness, and also the implacability of the tensions in their marriage. For how could a marital relationship be normal when the partners lived in a hospital? How could the relationship between siblings have the usual give and take? And how could a home be normal when it had been turned into a hospital?

"I know," Fred had said when Daniel told him all this. And just hearing that "I know" helped, for Fred really did know. He had been in so many of what Daniel called the "home hospitals," apartments or houses filled with hospital beds, walkers, rehabilitation machines, breathing equipment, and hospital linens.

For all the eleven years of their strange life since Sarah's first operation, Fred had been the one person he could call at any time, the one mind besides Lila's that could share his pain, and the only mind that could answer his questions.

But even Fred, Daniel feared, might be running out of answers.

"You think too much," Fred had said on the phone just a few weeks ago, in answer to one of Daniel's inquiries about what would happen next.

"That's a rabbi's job," Daniel replied.

"It's a doctor's, too, but look at me. I'm stupid."

The remark, delivered in Fred's offhand, sardonic manner, was a reference to his childhood, when Fred was considered the intellectual black sheep of his highly educated family.

"Some black sheep," Daniel thought, getting up and stretching his legs. Well, some firm answers would be coming from Fred soon, whether or not Daniel wanted to ask the questions. Lila didn't seem to be as afraid of the answers as he was. Indeed, she was anticipating them.

"This will be Sarah's last hospitalization," she had said tremulously as they walked through the hospital door, a few steps behind the wheelchair in which their daughter was being pushed.

"Fred will think of something," Daniel replied.

"No. He can't think anymore," Lila countered. "He's been trying to tell you that."

Resignation was written on her face, she who had fought for her daughter like a tigress, matching Fred's aggressiveness step for step. Before each operation, she would listen impatiently as he explained the risks.

"Will it help if you do it?" she would ask.

"I think so."

"Then shut up and operate."

Daniel looked at his sleeping wife and daughter, one the victim of exhaustion, the other victimized by a killer she had held at bay all her life. Fred's operations suddenly seemed like futile attacks on a dragon. You cut off one scale and another grew and then another. And always there was fire breathing out of the dragon's mouth. Yet somehow the maiden got rescued; he had to believe it would happen again.

Saint Fred and the dragon. Daniel in the lion's den.

Daniel walked down the dimly lit hall toward the nurses' station, where he was a familiar figure. Over the years, Daniel the persistent questioner had learned a lot about nursing. He knew, for example, that there was more paperwork than most people realized. He knew why it was difficult to be a "floater," to go from floor to floor when the hospital was understaffed. And he knew how important a kind word from a nurse, a note of reassurance, could be to a family's emotional well-being.

"We doctors go home, but the nurses are always there," Fred had commented more than once. Fred might provide the spirit that made everyone call the unit "Camp Epstein," but it was the nurses who gave the place its living soul.

"Coffee, Rabbi?" a nurse asked, directing him to the coffeepot kept on hand especially for parents.

Daniel shook his head and continued toward the soda machine near the elevator.

The elevator door opened and the Dagners emerged from a crowd of interns, the floral pattern of Ina Bea's dress contrasting starkly with the whiteness of the interns' uniforms.

"Dr. Epstein will be operating on Kevin tomorrow," Clayton Dagner said to the rabbi, trying to keep his voice as calm as possible.

There were two black Naugahyde couches on the wall facing the elevator. Daniel motioned for the Dagners to sit down, and he listened as they went over what Fred had told them. Kevin's tumor was an astrocytoma, probably not malignant, and Fred thought Kevin had a good chance of a complete recovery.

As they talked, Daniel's computerlike mind called up the file name "brain tumors," subtitled "gliomas," the general term for tumors that arise from the supportive tissue of the brain. It was a file he had steadily built up over the years.

A brainstem glioma, he knew, was usually an astrocytoma, sometimes an ependymoma, or perhaps a combination of the two. The tumor could be low grade, as Kevin's seemed to be. It could also be an anaplastic astrocytoma, which is mid-grade, or a glioblastoma multiforme, which is high grade and one of the most malignant and difficult tumors to treat.

So Kevin had "lucked out" in a way, if there was such a thing as luck when it came to tumors. Fred was hopeful that the tumor could be cured.

And why not hope for Sarah? Why not my beloved baby, after all these years? Because hers was the wrong category of tumor, Daniel reminded himself, the malignant kind, the kind with the dragon's scales. Daniel caught himself up short, realizing that he was jealous of the Dagners. "Tumor envy," he thought wryly. "Something new under the sun."

"If Fred says it will be all right, it will be all right," he told them, and inwardly he repeated the words over and over, like a mantra. In Daniel's mind, Fred could do anything, had to be able to do anything, so please God, let him be able to make it all right for Sarah, too.

Daniel's reassurance relieved Ina Bea for a moment; then he saw the terror gripping her again. Tears began to cloud her eyes. Daniel recognized that familiar flash of eternal guilt. He had seen it so many times, and it was constantly in his own head. Why did it happen? How? Could I have done something differently?

"Kevin had these headaches," Ina Bea said. "And I knew there was something wrong. But I didn't know what kind of doctor to take him to. And all the while, that tumor was getting worse. I should have . . . ." The floodgates opened, and the tears flowed.

"You mustn't blame yourself," Daniel reassured her. "There's no reason for it. It's simply rotten luck."

Did he really believe that? While taking part in a church service one Brotherhood Week, he had heard a sermon by a minister who had recently lost a son in a plane crash. "It's not a question of 'why' bad things happen," the grieving father had said. "It's a question of 'when,' and 'when,' it seems, doesn't get around to everybody."

That assuaged the guilt somewhat, put it all on the level of a metaphysical baseball game where everyone would strike out eventually, but somehow not everyone got called up to bat.

No. Daniel couldn't banish the question of "why." Didn't want to really, although he realized it was a question that couldn't do any good.

Gently, he advised the Dagners to go back to the hotel JoAnn had arranged for them and get some rest. "Rest" was a silly word in these circumstances, but it was the only one he knew. Ina Bea and Clay looked like the kind of small-town couple who couldn't get a good night's rest in New York City under any circumstances, much less the ones they now faced.

"We're going to spend some time with Kevin first. Tell him

as much about it as we can," Ina Bea said. She stifled a sob, and Daniel reached out and took her hand.

Daniel watched the Dagners walk down the hall, and saw them pause to glance into Sarah's room, which was next door to the room Kevin shared with Luis Olmedo. Clay Dagner put his hand on his wife's shoulder, as if to steady her, and his own back slumped a little.

Daniel realized that Sarah's appearance must be shocking to them. He remembered their stunned silence when they stopped by her room this morning to introduce themselves. Sarah's head was bent to one side, with her mouth gaping open and her face puffy from steroids, prescribed to reduce intracranial pressure. Her legs and arms were almost useless. She could move her arms one at a time, but only by dint of great effort, the effort she used to type on the computer. Her brown hair lay limply over her forehead, and her soft white face was frequently contorted by muscle spasms.

They're wondering if this is what their son will look like, Daniel thought. They're wondering if they'll be able to take it, how we've been able to take it.

We've taken a lot, but we've been given a lot, too, he wanted to call after them but thought better of it. The Dagners couldn't possibly understand. Not yet.

They couldn't know all the joy Sarah had brought. They hadn't seen her proudly riding a bicycle down the street, after four months of struggling to learn how. They hadn't been there when she helped him make a cake for Naomi's birthday, her shaky hands dropping more flour on the floor than in the bowl, but still they'd produced what Naomi pronounced "the Super Bowl of cakes."

And lately, after Sarah had become aphasic and couldn't speak, but amazingly could still sing snatches of songs, he'd joined her one Sabbath in her favorite Hebrew melody. *"Hiney*

mah tov oo mah nayim, sheveth achim gam yachad," they sang,
Sarah chiming in only on the last phrase, but loud and clear.
"How good it is for brothers to dwell together." For families
to dwell together.

Daniel felt the tears well up. His throat was dry, but he
realized that he didn't want to buy a soft drink from the
machine, his reason for coming down the hall in the first
place. No. He wanted to stretch out in that torturous chair
in Sarah's room and close his eyes, just for a little while. He
wanted to shut down his brain.

The sky outside had grown dark by the time Fred Epstein
arrived on Nine East. He had adopted the habit of making
early-evening rounds from his mentor, Joseph Ransohoff,
M.D., director of neurosurgery.

"Dinnertime. That's when most parents are there, and you
get to talk to them," Joe Ransohoff had declared when Fred
was his resident more than two decades ago. Many physicians
made rounds in the early morning, preferring to avoid facing
parents and their endless questions, but Ransohoff welcomed
them. Fred had absorbed this bit of wisdom and so much
more—knowledge, technique, self-confidence—from Ransohoff, a grand master.

Fred had originally planned to be a psychiatrist, like his
father and older brother, until his third year in medical school
when he was assigned to neurosurgical service for a month.
He made rounds with Dr. Isidore Tarlov, the neurosurgeon
in charge, watched him operate, and became fascinated by
neurosurgery.

Ransohoff had warned him off. "Being a brain surgeon isn't
like being a shrink," he insisted. "A shrink just thinks he's
inside the patient's head, but a brain surgeon really is. It can
be pretty scary in there, too."

But Fred knew what was right for him. He had proved to

be an ambitious and daring apprentice, eager to surpass his master. Ransohoff, for his part, welcomed the challenge, giving Fred plenty of room to try out new ideas.

It was Ransohoff who had supported the creation of the division of pediatric neurosurgery in 1985 and appointed Fred its director, but he refused to stand back as much as Fred would have liked.

Over the years, the pair had developed a love-hate relationship, and Ransohoff was one of the few people who could incite Fred to lose his temper.

Perhaps their arguments were occasioned by differences in personality, Fred subdued and reining in his emotions, Ransohoff following the grand tradition of the iconoclastic neurosurgeon, given to cursing, tossing instruments about in the operating room, and frightening residents—the doctor as macho man. He even had a tattoo on his arm.

Now in his mid-seventies, Ransohoff had recently become a father, and he was still as trim and muscular as a marine sergeant. He stalked the corridors in a pair of well-worn cowboy boots.

Fred had always thought that he and Joe Ransohoff were as different as day and night, until one of the nurses, dabbling in a bit of amateur psychology, pointed out that he, Fred, had started to wear boots too, reflecting perhaps a desire to be in Ransohoff's boots.

"Perhaps," Fred acknowledged, but the truth was, he had unusually high arches and regular street shoes hurt his feet. The ostrich-skin boots were comfortably loose, like his OR clogs, and for someone who was on his feet fifteen hours a day, comfort was a major issue.

Fred looked down at the list Tania had prepared for him of patients to see. "Barbie Marting, room 904," he read.

Fred had operated on Barbie, now six years old, three

years previously. During the operation, he had installed a shunt to drain off the excess fluid that had accumulated in her brain. Afterward, fluid continued to accumulate, so the shunt was left in place, as it sometimes is with brain tumor patients.

A shunt is actually a catheter, a narrow piece of tubing, which is inserted into a ventricle—one of the four cavities of the brain through which cerebrospinal fluid circulates—threaded under the scalp toward the neck and then on to another body cavity, where the fluid is drained and absorbed.

The development of the shunt a few decades ago is one of the medical advances that has increased the long-term survival of those with congenital hydrocephalus as well as the 10 percent of patients whose brain tumors block the pathways that permit cerebrospinal fluid to drain normally. Prior to the shunt's invention, there had been no effective way to relieve the abnormal accumulation of cerebrospinal fluid.

Many methods were tried unsuccessfully, including in the nineteenth century wrapping the patient's head in a tight bandage. Fred had tried to update this method in the 1970s, but even though Ransohoff gave his support and encouragement to the controversial idea, the experiment proved a failure.

Shunts, useful as they are, can still malfunction. Sometimes a catheter becomes clogged or is made ineffective by the presence of an infection. Then the patient feels nausea or suffers a headache, and sometimes experiences vomiting, double vision, or clumsiness.

Sometimes there are no symptoms at all, just vague feelings on the part of a parent that something is wrong. Fred trusted those feelings implicitly, whether they applied to a shunt or to other matters. There would be fewer late diagnoses of brainstem and spinal cord tumors, he thought, if more doctors responded to parental intuition.

In Barbie Marting's case, however, there was no need to rely on feelings. She had been suffering severe head-aches and muscle spasms, and her nervous mother, barely out of her teens, wanted to have the problem treated by Fred rather than by a surgeon in her hometown of Paterson, New Jersey.

"Barbie sobbed the entire time in the car," Mrs. Marting said anxiously as Fred performed his examination.

Barbie showed increased cranial pressure, signaling that the shunt was blocked or disconnected, which meant that she needed a replacement.

"I have an urgent operation scheduled for tomorrow, but my partner, Dr. Wisoff, will replace Barbie's shunt," Fred told Jennifer Marting.

Fred and his associates performed about three hundred shunt procedures a year, most of them on children with hydroceph-alus.

"I know you have to take care of the really sick ones," Mrs. Marting remarked, looking down at her daughter, who was crying from the pain. She couldn't know that Fred had another reason for adding Barbie to the schedule quickly. He was anxious to reunite the little girl and her mother with the rest of the family as soon as possible. The longer the separation, the greater the possibility of family dysfunction, particularly when the parents were so young.

"When are you going to take me, Doc?" came a strong voice from the next bed.

It belonged to twelve-year-old Jackie Holt, Barbie's room-mate, who was sitting up and glaring at him. With her usual eccentricity, Jackie wore a long white T-shirt with purple polka dots, the dots matching the purple tips of her punk hairdo. Makeup was piled on her face, since Jackie had decided that Nine East could use some "clownin' around."

Four years earlier, Fred had operated on Jackie for a low-grade astrocytoma of the brainstem, rather similar to Kevin Dagner's. She was here to check on some temporary symptoms—headaches and vomiting—but the tests, performed yesterday, showed no recurrence. More than likely, she simply had a virus. Still, Fred knew that Jackie, for all her bravado, worried about the tumor coming back. Worry was one of the legacies of having been a brain tumor patient.

"Hey, I'm not taking you anywhere, my friend, and you know it," Fred responded.

Jackie seemed to breathe a little easier.

"Too bad," she barked. "I really miss that old OR of yours."

The colorful getups, the strident style were Jackie's way of responding to the situation. Her more introverted mother had acted differently. At the time of Jackie's illness, she had withdrawn from her daughter, paying little attention to her and displaying no emotion. When Fred explained what he would do during the operation, Mrs. Holt stared at the wall. She asked no questions and merely shrugged her shoulders, as if he were talking about someone else.

Although this reaction was unusual, Jackie's mother was not the first parent in whom Fred had observed it, and Tania had observed it, too. She spent a great deal of time counseling Mrs. Holt, but the woman's withdrawal ended only after she realized that her daughter would live.

Fred suspected that Mrs. Holt retained a feeling of shame about her behavior, never looking directly at him if she could help it. During his interchange with Jackie, for example, she sat in a corner of the room, her eyes focused on her lap.

He went over and took her hand. "Jackie's okay. You know that," he said firmly.

Mrs. Holt offered him the beginnings of a smile.

"Give me a bigger smile," Fred urged.

"Come on, Mom, give the doc what he wants," Jackie echoed.

The smile improved, but the gaze turned downward again.

He squeezed her hand, then gave a quick squeeze to Jackie's shoulder as he left the room.

Fred only wished that he had some news that would make Lila and Daniel Glazer smile. They deserved it, for God's sake, he thought, and I deserve it, too. But we don't always get what we deserve in this life. His own mother, for example, a psychiatric social worker who had employed her brilliant intellect in the service of others, now suffered from Alzheimer's disease, unable to remember her own name. Still, his mother had lived a full life span, about seven times the years he had been able to give Sarah.

Fred found Lila and Daniel sitting by Sarah's bedside. The child, propped up by pillows, waved a wobbly arm at him, while Daniel looked at Fred nervously. Lila's cool eye met Fred's with an expression that said, "Go easy on Daniel."

All right, Fred thought to himself as he eased into the room, start off slowly, pal.

He moved Sarah's computer in order to examine her, then slid it back toward her. When he glanced down at the screen, he saw that she had typed the word "Hello."

"Hello to you. You know, Sarah," he confided, "I was so impressed with what you can do on the computer that I bought a laptop. I'm teaching myself to type."

Sarah fixed him with a stare. With great effort to keep her arm muscles under control, she reached for the keyboard, wrinkled her brow in concentration, and painstakingly tapped out "How fast?"

Fred leaned over and typed "Not as fast as you." The child gave him a lopsided grin before sinking back on the pillow and closing her eyes.

Sarah had been real tired today, Lila reported, so tired that she wasn't acting like herself. Usually, she refused to be given a shot in her own bed, insisting that she be moved to an empty bed for the procedure. She didn't like to have her bed turned into a "shot bed," she said. But today she'd taken an injection meekly without suggesting a move, even though the nurse was prepared to comply. Lila didn't have to add that the fight seemed to be going out of her daughter. Fred could tell by Sarah's groggy appearance, her diminished vital signs, and the notes on the nurse's chart indicating increased fluid accumulation.

"Let's take a walk, Daniel," Fred suggested.

In an empty room across the hall, Fred explained that he would be discussing Sarah's case at the tumor board, and he expected to be greatly influenced by the board's opinion.

Daniel seemed to regard the board as just one more consultation, a process to which Fred was more open than many specialists. Fred never acted hurt or insulted when worried parents wanted to obtain another opinion, feeling that they were entitled to whatever type of support they needed.

Now, Daniel observed, Fred was turning to his colleagues himself.

"That's true," Fred concurred, "but I have to tell you that you might not like what they tell me." He reviewed Sarah's numerous operations, emergency procedures to control bleeding, and chemotherapy treatments.

"Daniel," he remarked gently, "you and I both knew that this couldn't go on forever."

Daniel peered at him, his shining black eyes, sharp nose, and high cheekbones giving him a hawklike appearance. Fred stepped back uneasily, feeling as if he were being dissected.

The glare persisted. "I'm sure that you and the board will find a solution," Daniel said emphatically.

This wasn't the Daniel he knew, the Daniel who leaped to debate every side of an issue, who lusted after truth. This was a frightened father, closing off his mind from pain. As Fred watched, Daniel seemed to sink inside himself, as if he were covered from head to toe with a large prayer shawl. The shawl had Fred's name written on it.

"I'm not God," Fred wanted to shout. "Don't put me in that position." For the first time in their relationship, he wanted to steer clear of Daniel, yet he followed him back into Sarah's room.

Lila sat in an armchair, working on a needlepoint picture of a familiar subject: Fred being walked by his golden retriever, Chloe. Lila had flatteringly depicted Chloe as a much younger animal, replacing patches of hair that were long gone, and she had done the same for Fred.

Fred reflected that Lila, an expert needlewoman, had been working on the tapestry, intended as a gift to be hung over his fireplace, for more than two years.

"Hey, when am I going to get my present?" he asked. "It never seems to get finished."

"Soon, Fred, soon," she replied wearily.

"I tell her she has 'tapestry interruptus,' " Daniel joked. "It's a disease you doctors can't fix yet."

"No, they can't fix it," Lila said firmly.

She flashed Fred a look that went straight to the bone. He couldn't shake off the effect even minutes later as he sat next to Kevin Dagner's bed.

Kevin, who had been given pain medication, was resting

quietly, yet he was quite capable of carrying on a conversation. Fred's object was to tell the boy about the operation, but this had to be done cautiously. All children had questions, but some wanted to know more than others. It was a matter of finding out what was on Kevin's mind.

Fred drew the curtain around the bed so that the sleeping Luis Olmedo, Kevin's roommate, wouldn't wake up. Carmen Olmedo was waiting for Fred in the library upstairs, and Kevin's parents had left the hospital. Fred had the privacy he needed to talk to Kevin, and for developing his own relationship with the boy.

Because even the slightest movement of his face created agonizing pain, Kevin spoke slowly. He wanted to know why the tumor was giving him a headache, and what the tumor looked like. After Fred explained that the headache came from increased pressure on the skull, he took a pencil and a small pad out of his pocket and drew Kevin a sketch of the tumor, with its spiky edges.

Kevin considered for a while, then asked how Fred would get the tumor out.

"The tumor has gotten mixed up with other tissue in your brain," Fred said. "To get it out, I use an instrument, just about this size, that liquefies the tumor, sort of blowing it to bits, while keeping the good tissue safe. It's a little bit like *Rambo*."

Kevin smiled.

"I like that movie," he said.

Fred went on to explain that a portion of Kevin's head would be shaved for the operation. "But don't worry, we won't take too much," he said. "The soccer team won't notice." All kids worried about losing their hair—perhaps girls a little more than boys—and Fred and his staff made a real effort to keep the shaving minimal.

A nurse poked her head through the door. "JoAnn called to remind you that Mrs. Olmedo is waiting in the library," she said.

Fred nodded.

"Do you have any other questions?" he asked Kevin.

The boy tugged at his rumpled bedsheet, hesitant to speak.

"Well, it's not a question, really," he said after a time. "It's more like asking for something."

"Anything at all, Kevin," Fred responded, but Kevin's request would make him shudder. It reminded him why he rarely saw children this close to surgery, preferring to develop some emotional distance.

"Please don't let me die," begged the ten-year-old goalie.

CHAPTER 5

As Fred walked toward the converted storage space that served as a library and conference room, he thought of how important it was to persuade Carmen Olmedo to go on fighting for Luis's life. He already envisioned the second operation. In his mind, he was in the OR, peering down at the boy's spinal cord through the operating microscope, preparing to dispel the returning invader.

It wasn't that the recurrence was unexpected. Luis's spinal cord tumor had been malignant—a rarity for such tumors—and malignancies almost always return. Yet the sight of the growing tumor on the routine MRI had come as a shock.

So soon, Fred mused. He had hoped for more time, hoped, though he wouldn't admit it, for a cure.

Yet it didn't take long for him to make a surgeon's transition from disappointment to determination. He would just have to fight harder, and the boy's sociological circumstances fueled his commitment to employ every weapon in his arsenal.

"Luis lives with his parents in a slum that is subject to harsh flooding," Donald Brickelmeyer had written in his referral letter. "His grandmother and four siblings live with him. The house is made of cane and wood scraps, with a dirt floor, built on stilts. Poor drinking water quality and poor sewage. Garbage piles up everywhere."

The words of the clinic director were dispassionate, but to Fred they pulsated with meaning: "Save this kid. Even the score."

Fred's mother, a dedicated social activist, would have interpreted them the same way. At the Epstein dinner table, impassioned talk of social justice had been a standard part of the evening fare, and that memory was one reason why Fred sometimes absorbed the costs of treating underprivileged patients.

Alzheimer's disease had robbed Lillian Epstein of the ability to communicate with her son, yet Fred felt she was communicating with him now, urging him to be aggressive. He didn't need such a message, though. Already his fingers itched to grasp the Cavitron and unleash its powers of destruction and healing.

He was so deeply engaged in thoughts of surgery—had the scan shown all of the tumor? how much would he be able to get out?—that he sat down at the conference table without looking around him.

Lourdes Suarez, the nurse from the Dominican Republic who would act as translator, broke through his reverie with a quiet greeting and a shy smile. But Carmen Olmedo, Luis's mother, offered only a formal nod. Fred's stomach tightened as he noticed the way she was sitting, massive arms folded across her chest, eyes focused straight ahead. It was a stance designed to hold off outsiders, for even though Carmen was grateful to him for trying to cure her son, Fred knew that she still considered him an outsider.

Unlike most other parents, Carmen didn't share her feelings or welcome his expressions of empathy. The situation made

Fred uneasy—he preferred parents to be partners in treatment—but he realized that Carmen was as uncomfortable with
high-technology medicine as he would have been with the
herbal cures and remedies that constituted "medicine" in the
village of her birth.

Start slowly, Fred said to himself. Explain it all, bit by bit,
the way you did when you first met her. She may live in a
shack with five children and no running water, but she's smart
enough. Somehow she found the clinic that Don Brickelmeyer
runs, and she saved her son's life. She'll save it again, if I talk
to her right.

"The tumor has begun to grow again," Fred declared, trying
in vain to make eye contact. He explained that the recurrence
had shown up quite clearly on the scan.

Carmen seemed to be listening with interest, but her folded
arms remained stiff, as if to ward off his next words.

"The pictures show that Luis needs another operation,"
Fred went on. *"Un otra operación necesidad,"* he added, unaware that he had used the wrong article.

Lourdes corrected him with a smile, then put her hand on
Carmen's arm. If anyone could get through to Carmen emotionally, it was the young nurse, who came from a crowded
urban area not so different from Carmen's own. Her grandfather's small plot of land in the country had been sold to
send her to nursing school, with the understanding that she
would go to work in the United States and send money home.
Lourdes hadn't seen her family for several years.

"You can't imagine how strange everything is to her here,"
Lourdes had once told Fred when he remarked on Carmen's
reserve. He noticed the pain in her voice and realized she was
also talking about herself.

Now Lourdes's soft tones took on a compelling quality as
she translated his words, like a cloud with underpinnings of

iron. She's making her voice tell Carmen that she has to trust me, Fred thought, she's fighting to deliver my message.

Carmen allowed Lourdes to continue holding on to her arm, but she shook her head, unable to understand why Luis needed another operation.

"He has no pain," she pointed out.

In that, she was correct, for as yet a slight limp was the only physical evidence of the growing tumor.

"Luis will be in pain and as much as before if I don't operate," Fred went on. "The more quickly we treat him, the less pain he will feel."

There was a long silence, during which Carmen seemed to withdraw even further into herself. Perhaps she didn't believe what he was saying. Perhaps she was thinking about the first operation and the uncomfortable recovery period, when Luis had been given a long course of chemotherapy.

It was difficult to face all that again, yet the surgery and the therapy had extended Luis's life for three years. Fred believed he could give him more time, if only Carmen would cooperate.

But she dashed his hopes. "No operation," she announced with finality.

Fred battled hard against feelings of annoyance, the most negativity he would consciously allow himself to experience against a parent. Carmen Olmedo was thwarting his deepest passions: the need to get deep within the troubled tissues and extricate the killer, the need to make a child better through surgery. For an instant, his sympathy for her became clouded, and he found it difficult to maintain his easy air of amiability.

It was unusual for Fred to flounder as he felt he was floundering now. He glanced at Lourdes, seeking her assistance with his eyes.

He knew how much the nurses loved Luis, who was as

affectionate and open as his mother was controlled and re-served. One of Luis's favorite tricks was to throw his arms around a nurse's neck and hang on for dear life, giggling and snuggling close. Lourdes was particularly fond of "the little bear . . . *osito,*" as they called him, and sometimes smuggled in his favorite food, empanadas, because he called the hospital food inedible, and Lourdes secretly agreed.

Lourdes spoke a few words to Carmen in a firm voice.

"I told her that if you don't operate, Luis will die," she said.

"Tell her again."

Fred noticed beads of perspiration on the nurse's forehead, but Carmen became even more glacial and shook her head repeatedly from side to side. Fred feared that she would leave the room.

There was one last chance—if he could impress on her the advances in treatment and the many new options available since Luis's first operation.

There were new combinations of chemotherapeutic drugs, and new ways of administering them, through an artery, for example, or a cavity in the brain, or by implantable, biode-gradable pumps.

Research, too, held great promise if he could keep Luis alive long enough to benefit from it.

Scientists were trying to find ways to bridge the blood-brain barrier, which prevents many substances, including chemo-therapeutic drugs, from entering the brain and the spinal cord through the blood vessels. They were also studying mono-clonal antibodies, or MAB, which are manufactured by the body's white blood cells to fight off foreign substances or an-tigens.

The body regards tumor cells as antigens, and because an antibody binds only to a specific antigen, it can identify a tumor cell. MAB currently are being manufactured in the laboratory, using genetic engineering and cloning techniques. Eventually, they may be used to fight tumors.

How to explain such twenty-first-century concepts to a woman who lived, at best, in nineteenth-century conditions? Fred pared down the facts as best he could, and he could hear that Lourdes was choosing her words with care, making the translation as exact as possible.

He looked at the two women, one his ally, the other a momentary adversary—both coming from a world he could only guess at. He had been in the home hospitals of many patients, but he hadn't been inside Carmen's shack. If I lived there, would I trust me? he asked himself. The thought made him ashamed of his annoyance and renewed his natural sense of empathy. It was important to make a parent think you liked him or her, even if you were momentarily upset. Remember that, Fred, remember.

"Believe me," he urged, "Luis is dear to me. I made him better before. I think I can do it again."

For a moment, her brown eyes seemed to soften as she considered his words. But then some mechanism he didn't understand took over, and he could see her dismissing them. The veil came down with a vengeance.

"Believe me," he begged.

"No more operations," Carmen replied, and Fred's world came crashing down.

There was a sound of sobbing in the room as Lourdes Suarez put her face down on her arms.

"I'm sorry, Fred," she said, quickly composing herself. "That was unprofessional of me."

"No," Fred replied. "It was very professional. It's when you stop having those feelings that you're in trouble."

A few minutes later, he was alone, after asking Carmen

Olmedo to think at least about what he had said. She nodded yes, the most cooperation he had gotten since they began to talk.

He tried to put his emotions in order, reminding himself that the parent was the major decision maker, and that Carmen Olmedo had a perfect right to say "No more," if that was what she was saying. Some parents wanted him to come on with all guns blazing; others did not, but not many. Fred was tormented by the idea that Carmen really hadn't understood him.

He knew how attached she was to Luis, whose bedside she rarely left and whom she addressed repeatedly as *mi bebé*, "my baby." Sometimes, when she thought he might be cold, she would double up his blanket and wrap it around him, Indian-style, so that only Luis's dark eyes were visible. Then she would hold him in her arms and croon a lullaby to send him to sleep.

Was she really ready to give him up? How terrible if Luis had to die because Fred had failed to communicate clearly.

Whenever Fred operated, he groaned repeatedly to himself, an ancient sound that dispelled his tension. "Some people breathe deeply, I groan," he told whatever resident was brave enough to comment on the sound.

Now he was groaning again, running through all the surgical moves he would like to make for Luis—and would make tomorrow for Kevin Dagner. He could imagine himself in the operating room, could feel the strong lights on him, could hear the quiet, regular hum of the monitors.

Fred's genie, his passion for surgery, had been unleashed, and there was no pushing it back into the bottle. Everything else in the world vanished, hunger, fatigue, the commonplace noises of the hospital, and any appointments he might have. Fred Epstein was on his own planet.

He went back to his office and began to work on the plan for Kevin Dagner's operation. He examined Kevin's MRI pictures in the viewer and reviewed the work-up report. "Scan shows enhancing lesion in posterior fossa." Even though two tumors might be in the same place and classified similarly, each required an individual plan, based on the most minute differences and taking into account the aspects most likely to create danger.

Fred worked much longer than he intended to, his fervor fueled, if anything, by Carmen Olmedo's rejection of treatment for her own son. Everything on the plan had to be exactly right.

One hour later, Kathy Epstein, standing in the lobby outside the Grace Rainey Rogers Auditorium of the Metropolitan Museum of Art, would wonder where her husband was, but not too hard. She had a fairly good idea.

CHAPTER 6

*T*he numbers on the digital clock read 3:30 A.M. when
Kathy Epstein woke up, reached out to touch her
husband, and found herself alone in their king-size
bed. Before falling asleep, she had been annoyed at having
to attend the lecture alone, but her usual sympathy toward
Fred had returned, and she longed to hold him close.

She wasn't surprised, though, that he wasn't in the bedroom. At best, Fred slept fitfully the night before he operated.
It wasn't the thought of a patient's death that kept him awake,
but the threat of paralysis, the worst outcome he could imagine
and one that haunted him increasingly as the minutes ticked
away toward daybreak.

There were signs that he had tried to relax: a plate of grape
seeds on the night table, a new mystery paperback missing
from the stack he kept near the bed. Fred liked mysteries
because they wrapped up puzzles neatly, unlike the puzzles of
his real world. But tonight, it seemed, even a mystery had
failed to get his mind off things.

He had apparently padded off with the book to the library,
from which the muffled sounds of a videotape could be heard.

Kathy could make out the theme of *Cosmos,* a TV program that Fred said was his favorite because thinking about the universe put his problems in perspective.

Kathy went to the kitchen of their spacious East Side apartment to get a glass of water. As she walked back into the bedroom, her reflection was visible in a Victorian mirror with a painted frame. Even in the early hours of the morning, and bundled up in a bathrobe, she would be called attractive: large hazel eyes peering out from beneath blond bangs, a turned-up nose, and a smooth, trim figure kept in shape by regular aerobic classes. The image was of a woman at least ten years younger than she actually was, and it belied Kathy's status as the mother of five children, ranging in age from three to twenty-one.

People who had just met the Epsteins often assumed that Kathy was Fred's second wife, the mother of only the two younger children, and though the thought amused Fred, he was always quick to dispel it. "All my children are from one marriage," he would say. "I'm lucky. Kathy's put up with me for twenty-seven years."

This was a significant statement from a man who valued the security of long-term commitment. Fred couldn't take the risks he took, move freely in the Cosmos of his own peculiar universe, without the bedrock provided by Kathy and the kids. It was an old-fashioned arrangement, but one that worked well for the Epsteins, stemming as it did from Fred's intense emotional vulnerability.

Fred had grown up in a close-knit but competitive family in the Westchester suburb of Yonkers. His parents, both professionals, had high academic expectations for their three sons, but Fred felt unable to meet them. He had difficulty learning to read, a problem that would be classified today as a learning disability, but which then produced strong feelings of shame in both the sufferer and his family. Consistently, his report cards showed poor grades. "What will become of Fred?" was a question frequently passed around the dinner table, along with the gravy for the mashed potatoes.

"I always felt I was disappointing them," Fred remembered, and it was always words that tripped him up.

One experience was firmly lodged in his memory. It happened at a dinner party his mother gave when Fred was in his early teens. Most of the guests were intellectuals or artists. The Epsteins numbered quite a few performers among their friends, and Fred struggled to keep up with the quick repartee.

Finally, he spoke up, asking one guest to explain his last remark.

"Fred," his mother broke in, although the man was patient enough about answering, "you either haven't been listening, or you're abysmally ignorant."

"What's 'abysmally'?" Fred asked.

The sound of laughter erupted around him, and he felt like sinking into the floor.

Just thinking about it made Kathy want to take him in her arms, to comfort the little boy who still remained inside.

By the time Fred got to college, he was a little surer of himself academically—he had attended a prep school where classes were small and teachers sympathetic—but he was still unsure socially, and very, very shy. To cover up, he developed an easygoing, joking manner that made young women view him as a pal, rather than the romantic figure he yearned to be. Just when he thought he was getting close to a woman, the relationship would fizzle, leaving Fred as puzzled and hurt as he had been when he couldn't understand the meanings of words.

"I was jilted by every woman I ever met before you," Fred once told Kathy. "They thought I was boring." What dopes they must have been, she thought, for even then Fred was tall, attractive, and athletic, and didn't conceal his fierce interest in the world about him. Hadn't those women been able to see that beneath his joshing manner and self-deprecating wit, he desperately needed love? Kathy had.

She actually knew Fred at the time, lived near him on Fire Island during the summer, but she was eight years his junior and, in the words of an old-fashioned novel, she "admired him from afar." A cliché, but it hurt Kathy as much as Fred was hurt by the rejections he got. She knew how sensitive he was.

Evidence of that was scattered around their bedroom, in the form of the sentimental Victorian valentines Fred had given her over the years. He collected the turn-of-the-century treasures and delighted in surprising her, hiding them throughout the apartment so she would come across them when alone. She might spot a touch of lace beneath her pillow or on the bathroom mirror. The valentines she didn't find, he would present to her in the touching but intense manner that belonged to him alone, becoming an adolescent again for just a second.

Surely that vulnerable nature must have been noticeable in college to the young woman he had identified only as "Rachel" and with whom he had been so much in love. Yet one night, Fred heard from Rachel the deadly words he had been certain she would never use, "Can't we just be friends?"

No, he wanted to shout, No. But as usual, he held it all in, too devastated to confide in anybody, too devastated to continue going to classes. Seeking the familiar and the secure, he returned home from the college in Massachusetts and completed his undergraduate work at New York University while living at home.

Fred finally rediscovered Kathy when he had just graduated

from medical school. He had been casually dating her older sister when he spotted Kathy in a shop on Fire Island, where the Epsteins and Kathy's family had summer homes. At first, he was impressed that "little sister" had grown into a beauty, but the relationship soon deepened. It wasn't long before Fred was telling her things he had never told any other person, particularly about his keen sense of ambition.

"It sounds sappy, Kathy, but I really want to make a difference in people's lives. And I want to be the best doctor there is, too. Is that asking too much?"

"Not for you," she reassured him, yet from the beginning she sensed that supporting his intense commitment would turn into a full-time job for her. A doctor's daughter herself, she knew what living with a doctor was like, or thought she did.

"I married you because you were the only woman who would have me," Fred had once said, in his self-deprecating manner. He might just as well have said that she was one woman who would help him have it all—a large and loving family, a comfortable home, and an unspoken permission to commit himself fully to his work.

It wasn't long before Kathy discovered Fred's propensity to bypass the nuts and bolts of domestic life. Shortly after they were married, when Fred was still a resident, she was stricken with the flu, unable to drag herself out of bed.

"What can I do to help?" he asked sympathetically. "Would you like some tea and toast?" She nodded her head painfully and fell back on the pillow while Fred went off, she thought, to the kitchen. He disappeared for what seemed to be forever, leaving Kathy to wonder exactly how long it took to boil a pot of water or push down the toaster button.

Forty-five minutes later, Fred returned to her bedside, carrying a small paper bag that contained a paper cup of hot tea and two slices of toast wrapped in wax paper. He had ordered up from the corner delicatessen.

Fred often told this story on himself, and everyone laughed, including Kathy, but she saw a larger truth in it. In so many areas, Fred "ordered up," leaving others, JoAnn Baldwin in the office and herself at home, to put the nitty-gritty details together.

It was she who planned the guest lists for the parties he agreed to give, organized the packing for family vacations, and supervised homework. He was the "fun guy," playing catch with fourteen-year-old Jason and roughhousing with the little ones, Joseph, six, and Benjamin, four. Otherwise, he was helpless.

Even in such a simple matter as running an errand, Fred messed up, either losing the list of items he was told to pick up, or getting sidetracked because he saw something in a shop window he wanted to buy for her. For himself, he hesitated to buy expensive items, with one exception: a Ferrari sports car, which he adored but hesitated to drive, fearing to look like a show-off physician. Mainly, what Fred did with the Ferrari was to talk about it, so that everyone in the hospital knew how much he loved the car.

The hospital. Kathy never asked Fred where his mind was when he forgot a family obligation because she knew: in that place. His intense absorption in his work had to be accepted rather than understood, but this didn't mean that acceptance came easily.

Sometimes, for example, Fred went too far. Like the evening he was late for their oldest daughter's high school graduation party.

"He promised, Mom," Samara kept repeating, and "Do you think he'll make it?"

By the time Fred showed up, Kathy's nerves were tuned to a fever pitch and she unleashed a torrent of shrieks, with the kids adding a backup chorus. For Kathy, who came from a family of screamers, it felt good to let it all out.

"You knew about this," she shouted. "I reminded you a hundred times. It wouldn't be so bad if you hadn't promised." Fred tried to apologize, but the kids and Kathy didn't talk to him for three days, the worst three days in all their years of marriage. By the third day, Kathy had cooled down and begun to imagine Fred being kept at the hospital by a patient just about Samara's age, a patient who would never have a graduation party.

She didn't remember when she broke the silence, or perhaps there had been no words. It was possible that Fred had let a valentine or some other gift express his feelings. All she remembered was falling into his arms and pressing her head against his chest.

"I'm sorry," one or both of them had said, and Fred made some sort of joke. After that he had tried, really tried not to let her down again, and Kathy tried not to take his no-shows so seriously, and that was where they were now—living with it. She was too smart to ask him to choose between her and his work; that would have opened both of them up to too much hurt.

It would be easier, Kathy thought, if Fred would let her carry some of his burden. But he kept so much inside, rarely talking about his fears, even though she knew how the nuts and bolts of his practice worked. It was the scary parts of being a neurosurgeon that he couldn't allow her to share.

"What does it feel like to operate on a child?" she had once asked, many years ago.

"I can't make you understand," Fred replied.

"Why not?"

He thought for a long time, then shook his head.

"Look, Kathy, you go into a luncheonette and you order a sandwich, right?"

"Right."

"Well, I do the same thing. The only difference is that twenty minutes earlier, I was inside a child's brain, hoping I could save his life. Being in the luncheonette is like a shock after that, as if I've come from the moon. I want to say to the counterman, 'Do you know where I've been?', but there's no way he can know. No one can."

Except, although he didn't say it, for the three other pediatric neurosurgeons who were his best friends and with whom he could release his feelings: Luis Schut at Children's Hospital in Philadelphia, Michael Edwards at Moffitt Hospital in San Francisco, and Harold Hoffman at the Hospital for Sick Children in Toronto.

I'm not a doctor, but I'm not the counterman either, Kathy wanted to say until she realized the meaning beneath his words. He needed her to stay in the luncheonette world, the place where people laugh and chat, order sandwiches, and make tea and toast. By being earthbound, she made it safer for him to journey to the moon.

Yet sometimes she had a glimpse of that journey. Once, for example, she had gone to a longtime patient's funeral because Fred was called into emergency surgery. Now it was her turn to listen to the eulogy, look at the parents' drawn faces, and receive from them the hugs and tears that would have been Fred's.

I can do this for him, she thought. Why doesn't he let me do it more often?

"It's not fair," she once complained to Fred when he insisted on being alone after an operation had gone badly. "We've been married for twenty-seven years. We're supposed to be here for each other."

"You are here, just by wanting to be," he answered, reaching out to stroke her arm. "But I need some quiet time, to think. I kept a kid from dying because I removed a tumor in his spine, and that was good. But in doing good, I paralyzed him for life. So the question is, did I really save him? Did I help?"

He held up one hand to silence her and gently placed a finger against her lips.

"I love you for wanting to kiss and make it better. But it doesn't change what happens, Kathy. It can't. Just give me some time. You know I'll bounce back. I always do."

He smiled at her and closed the library door behind him. For a long time, she stood there, her fingers touching the door.

The library was her favorite room in their large apartment. It was where the family congregated to talk, watch television, and play board games from a large and well-worn collection, which ranged from Candyland to Trivial Pursuit. It was a charming hideaway, made cozy by a dhurrie rug and a number of nineteenth-century antiques, including a child's sled that served as a magazine table.

On the wall above the fireplace, there was an empty space, which awaited the completion of Lila Glazer's tapestry.

Perhaps Fred was staring at that space now, thinking about Sarah Glazer and all the children he had saved, only to lose in the end. At three o'clock in the morning, the "real dark night of the soul," as F. Scott Fitzgerald called it, it was difficult to put things in perspective. Fred was probably remembering the details of every tragedy, and overlooking the triumphs. Don't forget about those triumphs, my darling, please don't forget—the ones you talk about on *Good Morning, America,* the ones that get written up in the popular magazines. Do you know how proud I am of you, how proud we all are?

She wanted to open the library door and say the words, but she knew better.

Instead, she walked down the long hallway, checking on the children, listening to their steady breathing. Hard to believe that her redheaded, angelic-looking Ilana was the same teenager who sometimes challenged her authority. "Why do you give in to Mom so much?" she'd complain to Fred, when he reluctantly supported Kathy on some disciplinary point or other. If it were up to Fred, Kathy thought, the kids would be spoiled rotten. He hated for anyone to be angry at him— a parent, a patient, a wife—but particularly his children, so he gave in to their demands whenever he could.

There was another reason for Fred's indulgence of his children, one of which most parents are blissfully ignorant. He had too often seen the terrible things that could happen to a child, and sometimes very suddenly: a blinding headache out of the blue, a seizure, even a stroke.

"You need to surround yourself with healthy kids to survive in this field" was how Jeff Allen, the pediatric neurooncologist who worked with Fred, had once explained his attachment to his family. They all hung on, these doctors, to their own children as if they were a miracle, and they were.

After a weekend at home, it was a wrench for Fred to return to his "other" kids, the pain-racked bodies and stricken faces on the ninth floor. Yet that was the world he had chosen, the one he took such pains to shield her from.

The tape had stopped playing, but the door of the library didn't open. Perhaps Fred had fallen asleep in his favorite plaid overstuffed chair, his long legs stretched out on the ottoman, his mind finally at rest. Kathy hoped that was the case.

A wave of fatigue overcame her, and she returned to the bedroom and climbed back into bed. She rolled over, clutched Fred's pillow case, and sniffed in his scent. As she lay there, the verse of one of her favorite valentines from him ran through her head:

> *Say, then, thou'll not forsake me,*
> *Bid me my fears dismiss*
> *Then will I dearly, fondly, love*
> *The author of such bliss.*

The sender of the original valentine had penned the words "quite true," under the verse, and Fred had added a picture of himself.

I'll always be there for you, friend and lover, lover and friend, Kathy promised as she drifted into sleep.

CHAPTER 7

Operating Room 11 on the sixth floor of New York University Hospital, Fred Epstein's favorite OR, was designed to hold the amount of equipment you might see in a scene from an old movie: an operating table, anesthesiology pumps and gauges, a table of instruments, and a few stools.

Now, thirty years later, the room, made even less spacious by the addition of a glass-enclosed viewing area, almost bulges to accommodate the accoutrements of a revolution in medical technology: ultrasound monitors, anesthesiology monitors, taping equipment, a TV screen, and a cart that holds lasers, drills, electric coagulating tools, and the Cavitron. In a corner, resting on casters and peering down on the scene, is the cranelike operating microscope, seven feet high.

In the hour preceding Kevin Dagner's operation, nurses and technicians, clad in shapeless blue scrub suits, moved deftly around the room, taking care to avoid the black, red, and yellow power cords that snaked along the floor.

A technician checked the monitors and made an important decision: which station to play on the transistor radio that sat in the corner opposite the microscope. He finally settled on a "mellow" station that was acceptable to everyone in the room, and the sad strains of "Don't Cry for Me, Argentina" floated forth, overriding the gentle hissing of the sterilizer.

How appropriate, thought Mike Wilson, the sixth-year resident who was scheduled to assist with the operation. Mike was still feeling low, smarting from a reprimand delivered to him by Fred Epstein two days ago, if reprimand was the right word. Fred always spoke so calmly, but Mike could tell when he was being shot down.

"Mike," Fred had asked, "did you order an antibiotic for the Elverson boy without checking with his pediatrician?"

Tommy Elverson, whose shunt had been replaced by Jeff Wisoff, had developed a slight infection.

"I guess I did," Mike replied. "It didn't seem that important."

"Hey, it was that important. We're a team effort here, pediatrician, infectious disease specialist—everybody. That's why parents bring their kids to a major medical center. We need lots of help, and we don't want to step on anyone's toes. Remember that."

Mike had muttered something and left the room, annoyed at first, but then he realized that Fred was teaching him a few basics, among them: In caring for a child, the most important thing is mobilizing the right people.

There was a lot more to medicine than the clinical stuff, even if most doctors wouldn't admit it. But Fred, in his quiet way, laid it all out on the table. Having papers published, giving talks, getting noticed, all these he encouraged his associates and residents to do, helping them with the effort if need be.

In return, Fred expected his subordinates, particularly his

residents, to pay attention, and Mike, who considered himself a go-getter, was determined to oblige.

I won't screw up again, he thought, with a twinge of nervousness. His part of today's operation had to go perfectly, even though an outsider might have considered it minor. But then, an outsider had never prepared a patient's skull for opening.

There were no minor parts of neurosurgery—every detail had to be performed perfectly—and Mike knew that each part entrusted to a resident represented an act of trust.

"You can't learn neurosurgery by watching," Fred had once said. Doing was the only way, but how much and when was a decision the master had to make, and a risk he had to take.

Mike chewed hard on a piece of gum and watched the scrub nurses, the ones who directly assist the surgeon, unwrapping stainless-steel microsurgical instruments—long-handled so the surgeon's hands would not obstruct his view through the operating microscope—and arranging them in just the order Fred required on a draped table called an "overhead table." Not all of the tiny instruments—there was a variety of scissors, forceps, nerve hooks, retractors, and suction irrigators—would be used, but they had to be in place and in perfect working condition. The slightest nick or imbalance would impair Fred's ability to work in the minuscule area where Kevin's tumor was situated.

Prominent among the instruments was a tweezerlike type of forceps, designed by Fred himself with a flat tip, which he used to hold back delicate membranes and expose the tumor without harming the tissue. The nurses dubbed the forceps "Epstein's Ferrari" because it was as sleek and subtle as Fred's red sports car of the same name.

Mike was wondering if he would ever get to see that car

when the doors swung open and Kevin Dagner was wheeled in on a gurney, drowsy from preoperative medication. In spite of the sedation, there was an anxious look on the boy's face.

"You're going to be fine, Kevin," boomed a baritone voice.

The voice, which belonged to Murray Canter, was familiar because the burly anesthesiologist had visited Kevin's room the night before and explained what would happen when he was "put to sleep."

Now Murray's salt-and-pepper beard was hidden behind a blue paper mask, but his presence was still reassuring. In spite of the pre-op sedation Kevin had been given, a battalion of butterflies was zigzagging around in his stomach.

The butterflies continued their flight as Kevin felt himself lifted up by several pairs of hands and placed on the operating table. He was aware of strong light coming from above, the tugging sensation of the IV line that had been placed in his right hand, and then he heard Murray's voice again.

"Kevin," he said, "I'm going to put something on your big toe. It won't hurt. It's called a pulsoximeter. It lets me check the amount of oxygen in your blood. And the tight thing you feel is a blood pressure cuff I'm putting on your arm."

Kevin nodded drowsily.

"Now I'm going to put the sleep mask on your face, just like the divers wear," Murray continued. "Remember? We talked about it. Just breathe in and out. You won't feel anything. You'll just fall asleep."

The mask supplied a mixture of nitrous oxide (known also as "laughing gas") and oxygen. Then Murray added inhalation halothane, an anesthetic offering rapid-onset and, even more important, rapid-reversal properties. The drugs took effect.

"He's under," Murray said quietly.

Murray attached electrocardiogram leads to Kevin's chest

to monitor heart activity. Then he lifted the boy's chin slightly, opened his mouth, and inserted the endotracheal tube, a plastic breathing tube, into the upper trachea. He taped the tube into place, then connected it to a respirator.

From this moment, until the surgery's completion six hours later, Murray would control Kevin's breathing, watching from behind a board of digital monitors for changes in body signs that indicated too much or too little anesthesia was being applied. Children respond to anesthesia with much greater sensitivity than adults, so it's a challenge to keep them pain-free without dangerously lowering blood pressure or interfering with breathing.

Blood loss is also a particular problem with children, since they don't have much blood volume to begin with. To monitor loss, Murray inserted an arterial line in Kevin's left wrist to measure blood gases, then injected a muscle relaxant into the IV line to paralyze the internal muscles during the delicate surgery.

Each person in the room performed quietly yet efficiently. This was a highly trained professional team, each member able to anticipate the other's next move.

As Murray worked, Mike Wilson cleaned Kevin's penis with an antiseptic solution and inserted a Foley catheter to drain off urine and monitor urinary output. He taped the boy's eyes shut to keep them from drying out as well as to prevent anything from getting in. Then he stepped back to observe the child and was impressed, as always, by the patient's total stillness and utter helplessness in the hands of the doctors and nurses. This was a Mississippi boy whose mother probably wouldn't let him go out hunting without his dad, and now she had to let someone else do his breathing for him.

"We'll take care of you, Kevin," Mike said under his breath.

He glanced at Rick Abbott, Fred's associate, who was responsible for the first part of the operation and who stood nearby, observing Mike carefully.

Rick's dark-haired, boyish looks belied his status as an expert neurosurgeon. And his contained manner was in sharp contrast to his associates, Fred Epstein and Jeff Wisoff, who tended to be more emotional. But even though Rick was less spontaneous than his colleagues, he too was an excellent teacher who gave patient, thoughtful answers to any questions Mike and the other residents might ask.

Murray came up behind Mike. "Let's turn him."

They gently rolled Kevin over on his stomach, taking care not to dislodge any of the tubes or the airway that had been taped into place. Before Kevin arrived in the OR, nurses had covered the stainless-steel operating table with a warm blanket and a foam cushion; the latter would prevent his body from developing pressure sores while immobilized. Now two pads resembling oversized jelly rolls were placed under his chest and shoulders to allow Kevin to breathe freely and to keep his venous pressure from rising. The boy's head was lifted into a three-pronged headrest and held firmly in place by a pin fixation device. Mike tightened the wing nuts so that Kevin's head would not move during the surgery.

"We're on, Kevin," Mike thought as a nurse handed him a razor. Mike shaved a three-inch strip of hair from the inion, the most prominent point of the back of the head, to the midpoint of the neck. This area would be the operating field.

He was careful to remove only as much hair as was necessary, since Fred always promised his kids that they wouldn't lose too much hair.

"Children can accept the fact that they're very sick more easily than adults do," he once told Mike. "They don't wonder or ask 'Why me?' But they do worry about their appearance. Going easy on the hair is the least we can do."

Once there had been a real hair disaster, and Mike was relieved to think that he hadn't been involved. Another resident had shaved the *payess*, or side curls, from the head of an Hasidic Jewish boy, and the parents were inconsolable. Not only were the curls required ritually, but their loss would also make the boy the object of much teasing. It took some time for Fred to soothe the boy's parents, and after that he made sure that his residents paid even more attention to head shaving.

Near the shaved area, Mike slicked down Kevin's hair with Vaseline to keep the hair from getting into the operating field and perhaps causing an infection, always a particular threat with brain surgery. Before the development of antibiotics, if a patient developed an infection, such as meningitis, he or she usually died, which is one reason why the mortality rates for neurosurgery then were so high.

To stave off infection, Mike swabbed the shaved area with Betadine for a full ten minutes, using pack after pack of gauze sponges. As soon as he finished with a sponge, he dropped it onto the drapes covering a pail. Throughout the operation, a scrub nurse would keep a count of the sponges to make certain that the total used and unused at the end of the operation matched the number in the room at the beginning. A similar count would be kept of instruments, the idea being to prevent any item, large or small, from being left inadvertently inside a patient.

Satisfied at last with his cleansing technique, Mike threw the last swab into the pail and cast a glance at Rick Abbott. It was time for both of them to scrub up for the operation.

While Rick and Mike were out of the room, Murray stayed

behind his screen of monitors, checking them and adjusting the flow of anesthetic. Kevin's vital signs remained stable. Two hours had passed since he was wheeled into Operating Room 11.

The two doctors spent ten minutes scrubbing and rinsing from fingertips to wrists, from forearms to elbows, using a stiff brush and antiseptic soap. They backed into the operating room with hands upraised to prevent the water from dripping back onto their fingers. A circulating nurse handed them towels, then helped each into a gown, tying it in the back. They slipped their hands into sterile brown rubber gloves, held out by the nurse, and moved back to the operating table.

Again, antisepsis. Mike painted the shaved area on Kevin's skull four more times, then surrounded it with a blue cloth drape and applied a plastic drape, impregnated with Betadine, that would adhere to the skin.

Whistling, "Don't Cry for Me, Argentina," even though the radio had long ceased playing it, he injected the scalp with a diluted solution of lidocaine. This would inflate the tissue and make it easier for Rick to get a clean cut.

Mike stood back and surveyed his handiwork, pressing his gloves on a moist sponge to clean them as he attempted to convey an air of nonchalance. Pretty good, if I must say so myself, he thought. Kevin's skull was ready to be opened, and Rick Abbott took an authoritative step closer to the table.

He looked at the scans of Kevin's head on the viewbox, studying once more the exact position of the tumor. He had of course reviewed the entire operating plan with Fred earlier.

"Knife," Rick said.

A nurse handed him a scalpel from the overhead instrument table, which, as the name implies, had been moved into place over the operating table.

Rick grasped the knife firmly and without hesitating made a clean incision, from the inion to the third cervical vertebra, through the fibrous covering of the skull.

To separate the muscle from the bone, Rick used the Bovie, an electric instrument that looks like a piece of steel one inch long and five millimeters wide and works with great speed. Connected to a small voltage unit, the Bovie can either obliterate blood vessels or burn off tissue, depending on the level of power used.

Working deftly, Rick stripped the muscles from the vertebrae at the base of the skull, exposing the bone.

"Retractor."

He inserted the retractor, which resembles scissors with long, curved, blunt blades, into the area to hold the wound open.

Then Rich asked for the perforator, a small stainless-steel air drill, and proceeded to bore a circle of burr holes, a half inch in diameter, in the bone around the exposed skull. Mike stood by, removing blood and tiny bits of bone with a suction device. As he dropped the sponges into the draped pail, the nurse continued to count them, and also to evaluate the amount of blood loss they evidenced. A craniotomy, the procedure Kevin was undergoing, could easily use up to sixty sponges.

Rick exchanged the drill for the rongeur, a pair of biting pliers used by neurosurgeons to chip away at the skull until they get the size opening they want. Rick worked steadily on the bone between the burr holes. Bone chips and blood clots flew out like bits of nail from toenail clippers, some of them hitting Mike's mask and sticking to his exposed eyebrows.

Damn, he thought, but he remained glued to Rick as if he were his shadow, irrigating the site and suctioning off the fluid.

Finally, Rick stepped back and looked at the opening, three inches square, that he had created.

"Bone wax," he said softly.

He dabbed the warm substance with his gloved finger around the burr holes to control bleeding, then coagulated exposed blood vessels with the bipolar unit.

"How are we doing, Murray?" Rick asked.

He was concerned about the effects of blood loss on Kevin's blood pressure.

"Okay."

Rick breathed a sigh of relief.

As he relaxed for a minute, three circulating nurses—who perform nonsurgery-related tasks—struggled to move the operating microscope nearer to the operating table.

It was hard for the nurses to suppress giggles as the monster machine, which they had just finished covering with sheets of sterile plastic, proved difficult to manipulate. Even with a nurse on each side clutching a handbar, the ponderous zigzagging scope seemed to have a mind of its own. Finally, they got it ready to be moved into place over the operating table, balancing weight facing the wall, dual eyepieces poised for surgeons' eyes, camera ready to be activated.

As they worked, Kevin Dagner lay hidden from view by layers of sterile drapes. The gentle sighs caused by the movement of the respirator were the one reminder that a living child rested on the table, waiting in sleep for the ultimate invasion. Now only the dura, the tough, shiny membrane that covers the brain, stood between the surgeon and intrusion into the organ itself.

Wearing magnifying glasses to enhance his vision, Rick, using first a knife and then scissors, created a Y-shaped opening in the dura. Blood gushed to the surface.

"Bipolar," Rick called for the coagulation unit. As he cauterized the cut blood vessels, Mike suctioned the area dry and packed Gelfoam—a substance that quickly absorbs blood—into the cavity.

The two doctors paused for a moment to see if the bleeding would stop. It did. Mike's heart stopped doing the slight flip-flop that was usual when it seemed that a "bleeder"—bleeding that had to be gotten under control quickly—might develop. He wondered if Rick was nervous, too, but nothing showed in the surgeon's eyes.

Experience probably does the trick, Mike thought. Rick had been Fred's associate for four years. A graduate of Baylor University Medical School, he had decided on neurosurgery during medical school, he told Mike, after watching an operation on a teacher suffering from a brain tumor. "A woman's life was transformed before my eyes," he said. "Here was a problem you could do something about. It was an exciting prospect."

Rick checked the bleeding one more time. Then, using a forceps, he lifted back the pieces of cut dura, patiently, one by one, and sutured each down with a prethreaded needle. He covered the pieces with strips of cottonoid, a gauzelike fabric, which Mike kept moist with saline solution from a syringe to prevent the dura from shrinking and making closing difficult.

Mike also suctioned the area, eliminating any remaining blood. The sound was not unlike that of a young child finishing a bowl of soup or slurping up the last bit of a milkshake through a plastic straw.

The sounds may have seemed less than medical, but Mike's actions were not. Every step he took was exactly the way Fred himself would have done it. "A resident has to be an extension of me," Fred once explained. "If you do anything so much as a millimeter differently, even the way you suction, it's a different operation."

Mike watched Rick carefully, absorbing every bit of his technique—which was also Fred's—and itching to try it himself. Soon, he thought, Fred will let me do more soon.

Finally, the last bit of dura had been peeled back. Kevin Dagner's brainstem, fully exposed, appeared to pulsate like a tiny heart, due to the blood vessels that fed it. It was difficult to believe that the source of Kevin's ability to breathe was housed in this tiny bit of tissue.

The doctors and nurses stared, as if they had never seen a brainstem before.

"It's always a wonder," Rick commented, in part for the edification of the visitors who watched from behind the glass window.

"Yes," Mike agreed.

No one spoke for a moment, then Rick cleared his throat.

"Tell Fred we're ready for him." More than three hours had passed since Kevin Dagner was wheeled into the OR.

One of the circulating nurses walked over to the wall phone.

"Hello, JoAnn. You can tell Fred we need him now."

As the doctors waited, Rick and Mike kept their arms bent at the elbows, the classic position to prevent them from inadvertently contaminating their gloves.

Mike's shoulders began to ache a little, but he felt a renewed spurt of energy. He'd done well during the first part of the operation, he thought. Why, he wondered, had he been dwelling so long on Fred's reprimand? An attack of resident hypersensitivity, no doubt.

"See anything interesting on television last night, Annie?" Mike asked a nurse.

As she told him about it, she handed him the small blue

syringe. Mike gently bathed the cottonoid strips covering the flap with sterile solution, while the nurse checked over the instruments once more and recounted the events on her favorite sitcom.

The only other activity in the room was the flickering and soft beeping of Murray's monitors, tracking heartbeat, blood pressure, respiration, temperature, urine flow, and other vital data.

Everything was muted, in a holding pattern, and all the time, Kevin Dagner's brainstem, peeking out from drapes and coverings, continued to beat from the arterial pulse.

Suddenly the doors swung open, and Fred Epstein, dressed in blue scrubs, strode into the room on his favorite green clogs. The clogs, veterans of many operations, were as comfortable to Fred as a pair of well-worn athletic shoes would be to a runner. A circulating nurse helped him gown, then held out a pair of sterile gloves. Fred shoved in one hand at a time with so much force that everyone in the room could hear the elastic snap. Then he walked up to the operating table and looked down at the open cavity. "Well, now," he said, "let's see what we have."

CHAPTER 8

FRED

Are you a believer?" This question or its equivalent is often asked of me, and I answer: "In my business, you have to be a believer."

I'm not a formally religious person, but I do know that we are in the hands of a higher power, particularly at moments of greatest risk. "There are no atheists in the intensive care waiting room," a parent once told me. There aren't many in the operating room either, particularly among the surgeons in our risk-filled specialty.

Neurosurgery as a specialty is less than a hundred years old. The first professional society, the American Association of Neurological Surgeons, was founded in 1931 as the Harvey Cushing Society. Until fairly recently, neurosurgery was the surgery of final resort. Not many patients survived. It was difficult for a surgeon to find the tumor without causing damage, difficult to remove it without doing the same, and if the first two maneuvers were accomplished, difficult to prevent a fatal infection afterward.

A neurosurgeon was considered a "death doctor," the last hands to touch the patient before the undertaker. No wonder so many neurosurgeons developed bizarre personalities, ego-centric, eccentric, or both. When you constantly have to take risks that don't pan out, it's natural, it seems to me, to go a little bit over the edge.

I think about those pioneers often, and I wonder what they would think if they could see the equipment I have at my disposal today. What does he have to worry about, they'd probably wonder?

But the worry is always there, because the nature of the brain hasn't changed—and neither have tumors. They're still nasty and strange, particularly in the brainstem, where they always entwine with a functioning system, the delicate tissue that controls all bodily functions. You're dealing with micro-pathways that converge into cables just like the wires in a telephone receiver. There's no room for errors. Even with the best scans, I can't tell the full extent of a tumor or what problems there are going to be until I'm standing there, look-ing inside the open skull.

The opening in Kevin Dagner's skull was just large enough for me to work in—perfect. Rick Abbott had done his usual fine job, and from the piercing look that Mike Wilson was giving me over his mask, he wanted me to know that he had been intensely involved, too. Like most residents, Mike wanted to perform, to get ahead, just the way I had been and Joe Ransohoff before me.

I nodded my head toward Mike and asked the nurse for the forceps. With the forceps, I gently separated the cerebellar tonsils and exposed the rostral area of the tumor, the area in the region of the brainstem.

"Ultrasound."

A nurse handed me a tiny transducer that converts sound

waves, which are deflected and then converted to an image. Since the perfection of ultrasound about a decade ago, it's been possible to trace and measure a tumor, just the way obstetricians record the activities of a fetus. The surgeon no longer has to palpate the surface of the brain to estimate where to make an opening to keep from going through healthy tissue, or to hunt with his fingers through the forbidding folds of the brain, risking damage to normal tissue. I would use the ultrasound transducer intermittently throughout the surgery, not only to monitor the dissection, but also to identify residual cysts, if any, around the tumor. These cysts must be drained as the tumor is destroyed.

I placed the tiny transducer on the pulsating brainstem, its steady beat created by the arterial pulse, and an image appeared on the ultrasound monitor. I could tell that the tumor was located beneath the surface of the fourth ventricle of the brainstem, confined almost exactly to the area it appeared to occupy on the MRI.

That was a relief. I've had experiences where tumors turn out to be larger than they appear to be on the scan, and that makes it necessary to widen the cranial opening, thus increasing the operating time.

I removed the transducer and gently placed a small tube containing an electrode on the open brainstem. It would be used to relay signals of the electrical activity in the brain, called the "evoked potentials." There is a normal delay of less than a millisecond between the time an electrode transmits and the time the transmission appears on the monitor. If the delay lengthens by even a fraction, it means that the electrical activity between the tumor and normal tissue has become disturbed, probably because I'm coming dangerously close to the normal tissue. I have to stop doing whatever it is that's causing the trouble—and fast. There was also an electrode on Kevin's foot that monitored the level of muscle paralysis. If the paralysis became too severe, Murray would have to cut back on the drugs he was administering.

Like ultrasound, the ability to track evoked potentials is one of the advances that have made neurosurgery a whole lot safer in the past ten years.

However, the major advance is the operating microscope, developed forty years ago but not generally used until the mid-seventies, with its power to magnify the operating field up to twenty times. Like other neurosurgeons my age, I once did without the scope and relied on magnifying glasses, but now I can't for the life of me imagine how we did it.

Two nurses moved the scope into place over the operating table.

I used a foot pedal to lower the scope, ordered it turned on, then peered down through it at Kevin Dagner's tumor. At the same time, a duplicate image appeared on a television monitor at the side of the room.

The difference between the two images was that the one on the monitor was two-dimensional, whereas my view was three-dimensional, as if I were wearing 3-D glasses. I could see the bright red of blood vessels, the creamy white of edematous and bulging brainstem tissue, and the gray of the tumor as it insinuated itself downward, rather like marbling in a steak. I could see the top of the "steak" and the layers below.

I gently elevated the cerebellum, which partially obscured my view, in order to get an even better look at the mass.

Thanks to Rick's work, and to the power of the instruments around me, the tumor was almost completely revealed. Now it was up to me to "debulk" the tumor. This is a process in which I remove the tumor starting from the center, destroying it bit by bit, and leaving the surrounding normal tissue undisturbed. It's somewhat like coring an apple by starting inside instead of through the skin.

There was absolutely no margin for error. Other parts of the brain have backup systems; if one area is injured, another takes over. But that's not the case with the brainstem. What's destroyed remains destroyed.

"Let's get this on tape," I said.

A nurse activated the camera inside the scope, and the tape began to roll. My venture into Kevin Dagner's brain would be completely recorded for teaching purposes and for the medical record.

In the back of my mind, I always have the idea that I might see such a tape in court some day. Every surgeon has the same fear. My malpractice insurance costs almost $100,000 a year, and though I always level with parents about the risks, I have been sued. It's a shattering and humiliating experience. I told one family that the operation would probably leave their child with bowel and bladder problems. When this happened, the child's family went to court, claiming they never heard me say that.

So far, though, I've mostly been lucky when dealing with parents, and in this business, as the saying goes, it's just as important to be lucky as it is to be good.

I reviewed Kevin's case out loud, even though there was no audio to go with the tape: "This is a ten-year-old boy from a small southern town. His mom is a nursery school teacher; his father runs a hardware store. They love him a lot. He's an only child, and he plays soccer. Let's make sure he'll play soccer again."

Not a very scientific description, but in this way I gave my team a pep talk, and I mobilized myself, too. I remembered the frightened child who had suffered such pain, had begged me for his life, and I visualized his parents, waiting on the ninth floor, too anxious to move about, too uncomfortable to sit still for long. Only my report would provide release, and that report would depend on what was happening here, now.

"Please activate the laser, Annie," I said to a nurse. "On twelve watts, continuous."

She switched on the laser. Pressing the control pedal with my foot, my eye fixed on the spot through the microscope, I pointed the laser directly over the tumor.

The laser, which looks like a small wand, is the ideal instrument for making—burning, actually—an incision into a tumor through the floor of the fourth ventricle.

Anyone who has ever used a magnifying glass to focus the sun's rays to burn a hole in a leaf has some idea of how the laser works. It delivers the concentrated power of light under high magnification, literally vaporizing the tumor.

The trick with a laser is to create exactly the right amount of power, and getting it right is a matter of judgment, experience, and instinct—that old triumvirate. As I worked, whiffs of smoke rose from the wound.

"Cavitron."

I've been using the pencil-shaped, ultrasonic instrument since the late 1970s, and it's become an extension of my fingers.

Alternately, I applied the laser to the tumor, then the Cavitron, which vibrates at 23,000 times a second. The Cavitron liquefied the tumor and simultaneously suctioned it out through the hollow inside of the tip, depositing it in a receptacle some distance from the operating table.

As Rick gently moved a retractor along, we uncovered and destroyed the tumor, hidden, snakelike, within the brainstem. As we left each minuscule area, an identation might become visible where the tumor had existed just a second before, and occasionally a tiny pool of liquid appeared as a cyst was drained.

It was painstaking work. I had to hold myself back from moving too quickly, since I'm always eager to eyeball more and more of the enemy. Such passion is a two-edged sword in neurosurgery. It creates the energy that makes you daring, yet the energy must be kept under control. One tiny slip and you're pulverizing healthy tissue, damaging rather than healing.

Step by step, I tell myself. I talk to myself under my breath as I work, and I even talk to the instruments—"Be very careful, easy now"—but not too loud. My associates and residents put up with it, but must wonder sometimes, I'm sure. Everyone has his or her own way of dealing with nervousness, and talking and groaning are probably mine.

I think I'm relaxed when I work, yet there's a peculiar kind of tension underneath that's endemic to neurosurgery. If you're not in a special kind of agony, you can't be any good. If you let the agony overwhelm you, you screw up.

It's a delicate balance, but one I've learned to live with, and it puts me in a different dimension. I've tried to explain it to Kathy several times; but though no one knows my soul better than my wife, I can't take her to that other place with me.

Someday, I think, I'll look in the operating microscope and discover that nameless dimension all mapped out for me, the same way the scope maps out the tumor. Then I'll be able to understand it and share it without having it overwhelm me.

I exposed most of Kevin Dagner's tumor, and the inside was firm, without its own supply of blood vessels. Though only a pathology report would tell for sure, this was a pretty good sign that the tumor was benign. Malignant tumors tend to become vascular and, therefore, spongy.

"It's relatively avascular," I commented. "Mike, take a look here. See what the thing looks like."

Rick took hold of the retractor, which Mike had been holding, and let the resident peer through the second eyepiece of the microscope, "the teaching eyepiece."

It's aptly named, since teaching is a large part of a senior surgeon's job. A resident is someone to whom you're passing on your knowledge, so you have to explain everything you can, at each step of the way. Little by little, the resident learns to do one thing, then another, then puts it all together without realizing that he or she is doing so.

Almost everyone is teachable, I've found. A resident rarely has bad hands, only a bad head, and adequate supervision can usually instill a sense of preparedness.

Residents also need to learn more than the techniques of surgery. They need to realize that no surgeon is God and that there's no excuse for arrogance. They have to know that we can gain knowledge from one another. It's important to encourage others to disagree with you from time to time, to make suggestions as Jeff Wisoff and Rick Abbott often do with me. I try to teach residents to welcome new ideas, whether they come from a senior surgeon, a nurse, a student, or another resident.

When it comes to the performance of surgery, it's a judgment call whether a resident is ready to do something.

Once, during another operation, Mike was anxious to make the incision in the dura, but the brain was badly swollen and the tumor was pushing right against the dura. I didn't think he would be able to make the incision without causing injury. The dura is tough, but it's only a millimeter thick. Rather than telling him that he didn't have enough experience, I just said, "Let me show you some tricks to open the dura when a tumor's pushing against it." So I did the cutting, but with his eyes closely following what my hands were doing. Someday his eyes will become his hands and, by extension, my hands.

Now Mike and I examined Kevin Dagner's tumor through the microscope, looking for every trace of it.

Suddenly Murray's voice called out: "Fred, are you manipulating something?"

His monitor showed an irregular heartbeat as well as a wildly fluctuating blood pressure. I had to work quickly. There was less than a second to correct whatever was wrong.

"Rick, check the retractor," I said calmly.

He looked at the stainless-steel instrument with which he was holding back a tiny bit of tissue.

"I may have been pulling on something," Rick replied, loosening his grasp somewhat.

"This better, Murray?" Rick asked.

"Fine, it's okay," the anesthesiologist said.

There was a collective sigh of relief. We can't always tell what's wrong that quickly. Sometimes we just have to stop whatever we're doing and step back until we figure it out. *Primum non nocere*, Latin for "first do no harm," the classic rule of medicine, has been transposed into "stop yourself from doing harm."

The possibility of doing harm is always on my mind and, even worse, harmful things can happen to patients even though the surgeon has done nothing wrong. It's simply in the nature of the operations we do, in the nature of the brainstem and the spinal cord, with their lack of maneuverability.

I remember every patient who ever "went bad" on me. One who really stays in my mind is a boy from northern Italy on whom I operated twice for a spinal cord tumor. The initial operation went very well, and fourteen-year-old Marco, who was a skiing enthusiast, was able to hit the Alpine slopes within weeks of returning home.

Three years later, I operated on him again in exactly the same manner and this time, too, everything appeared to be fine. Yet in the recovery room, Marco was unable to move. After I got the call from my resident, who was with him, I raced to the room. I recall tickling the bottoms of Marco's feet over and over again to see if the reflex movement of the toes was normal. "I love you Marco, move for me, move for me"—but there was no response and several weeks later there was still no response.

Having to live through those weeks with his father was one of the hardest things I've ever done in my life.

Marco's tumor hasn't come back, and he's alive and well, but he's a quadriplegic. He still gets to go to a ski lodge every winter, but all he can do is watch the skiers from his wheelchair. I wonder what he thinks about as he sits there. I hope he's achieved some kind of inner peace, and I ask myself if I could.

There would have been no hope of Marco's surviving if I hadn't operated on his tumor, yet that fact is small comfort. If I can't make a patient better than he would have been without me, what am I good for? And I can hear my mother's voice, commenting sadly on my grades in school, "Did you try your best, Fred, did you try your very best?"

After that first "devastation," I told Joe Ransohoff, "I don't ever want to go through this again."

He blew a cloud of cigarette smoke in my face and looked me up and down.

"You will," he said.

And I did, and I will again.

There's one important consolation, though—in fact, the whole history of medical science is built upon it—we learn from our experiences, no matter how much pain they cause. Even if something goes wrong for no apparent reason, as it did in Marco's case, I try to find out if there's something to learn from a failure, and I tell my residents to do the same. It's the only way to make sure that a child hasn't been "devastated" in vain.

In Marco's case, I learned that no matter how smoothly a procedure seems to be going in the OR, the final outcome can be unpredictable. The bottom line is how the patient reacts later on.

I thought about that as we approached the final part of Kevin Dagner's operation.

"Any other problems, Murray?" I asked, picking up the Cavitron again.

"Nope."

Apparently, the monitors reflected no abrupt changes in Kevin's respiration or blood pressure, or anything else that was being minutely checked. All throughout the surgery, Murray had been monitoring Kevin's nerve activity, assessing the level of muscle paralysis, and also gradually lightening the amount of anesthetic. The lighter the anesthetic, the more easily the evoked potentials can be read. That's why Murray uses fewer drugs and more narcotics, less halothane than before, so as not to inhibit those readings. This was the time when those readings would be of the most critical importance.

"I'm going to do what I promised, Kevin," I thought. "I'm going to save your life."

The operating room is where I make the child mine. I honestly believed what I told myself; I always do. Otherwise there is no point in offering hope to parents, no point in living with myself. I'm the best at what I do, and I never operate thinking otherwise. There's a lot of agony to live with, but I couldn't live with the agony of thinking that someone else could do it better. What I do takes a strong ego.

The Cavitron moved again. As more bits of tumor vanished, I could see that the remaining part grew deep into the brainstem, deeper than the ultrasound or looking through the microscope had indicated. Until confronted in the OR, tumors are impossible to predict, and I'm never surprised when one is harder to work on than I thought it would be.

I was considering my options when blood started to bubble up in the operating field, like water from an underground sprinkler. A bleeder.

"It's getting pretty juicy in there," Rick said calmly.

A nurse handed him a small cottonoid, and he placed it carefully in the cavity. Within seconds, the gauze was bright red. Another cottonoid, and then more, the nurse's hands moving swiftly, and Rick's and my hands even more swiftly.

"Gelfoam."

Rick and I packed the area with the substance. Then we stood by, watching, waiting to see if the bleeding would stop.

"All bleeders stop eventually," a director of surgery once told a group of residents, of whom I was one. But how long is "eventually"? That's the question that can stop your heart when you're trying to be—indeed, must be—calm.

The waiting continued.

"If it doesn't stop, we'll go after it," I told Rick and Mike, meaning that I would expose that area more completely and cauterize it using the bipolar, a tweezerlike device in which the current passes only through the tip so that it can be carefully controlled. Simultaneously, we would use the suction device, a tube about one millimeter in diameter, to clear the area of blood.

Fortunately, the Gelfoam did the trick. The blur of red disappeared from the microscope, and the operating field became clear again, the tumor taunting and tempting me with its depth.

This was the moment of greatest decision: How much more of the tumor to take?

If a brainstem operation gets ruined, it happens in the last five minutes, when the neurosurgeon removes too much of the tumor. The key is knowing when to stop.

And it's terribly hard to make yourself stop. You're always pushing to do more, to be aggressive. A degree of machismo is involved, even though the brainstem is no place to play little-boy games.

Harvey Cushing, the brave founder of modern neurosurgery, posed the dilemma for all time: "When to take great risks, when to withdraw in the face of unexpected difficulties; whether to face an attempted enucleation of a pathologically favorable tumor . . . with the prospect of an operative fatality or to abandon the procedure short of completeness with the certainty that after months or years even greater risks may have to be faced. . . ."

Technology has advanced so much since Cushing's time that it's possible to remove far more of a tumor than he would have been able to, though the removal of a brainstem tumor is something he wouldn't have considered at all. Be that as it may, the basic problem remains the same.

I had debulked 80 percent of Kevin Dagner's tumor. My operating plan called for 90 to 95 percent, the optimum that can be removed of most brainstem tumors.

I decided to forgo the last 10 percent. Kevin's tumor, an astrocytoma, was of the slow-growing variety. There was a chance of recurrence, but I hoped that his immune system would destroy or hold at bay the remaining tumor. I had taken out the branch, and the remaining leaves might well wither.

Rick was looking at me, waiting to see what my decision would be. This wasn't a matter for consultation. Rick might have wanted to do things differently, but the operation had to follow my command.

"Let's irrigate and close," I said. "We've done our best."

He nodded, and so did Mike. I considered that both men, one topnotch, the other fairly green, were at different stages along the ladder.

With his cap pushed back on his head, Mike looked like a kid, but someday he would be as good as Rick and Jeff, and those two would eclipse me. It was an unnerving thought, because I like to be on top, and I'm propelled by a need to be there. Maybe that's why I put the words "PED-NS1," "pediatric neurosurgeon 1," on the license plate of my Ferrari.

I fear being overtaken, fear growing old. So sometimes I look at my associates the way Joe Ransohoff must have looked at me when I first came on his service, full of new ideas and aggressive as hell. I suspect he found me scary and stimulating at the same time—but to his credit, he decided to keep me around.

Who will keep me around when I can't command anymore or make the split-second decisions that count? I don't think about it much. I try to keep myself totally in the present, where life is rich and rewarding.

Watching Rick suture the dura and replace the fragments of bone that had been removed, I thought of my own kids, and about Kathy, who is with me at times like this more than she understands.

"Hey, Mike," I said. "Go to the recovery room with Murray, and let me know as soon as there's a response."

He nodded yes, glad to undertake the assignment.

I walked out of the OR and started to remove my gown. It would be an anxious time until I heard from Mike. Though I thought Kevin would be fine, I couldn't be sure until a neurological exam had been done.

Then I would know what kind of news I would have for the Dagners, and how I would give it to them.

CHAPTER 9

A short while before Kevin's operation was scheduled to begin, Ina Bea Dagner had stood at his bedside, watching her son struggle with his fear and with the returning pain.

"It hurts again, Mom," he said.

"I know, dear, I know. But Dr. Epstein is going to make it better, soon."

They were familiar words, words she had spoken all his life. "It will be better soon, dear," when Kevin fell off his bicycle, scraped his knee, or had a rare argument with a friend. But now those words sounded pointless, and terribly out of place. There was no reason for Kevin to trust them. They had proved their unreliability when Ina Bea used them in regard to their family doctor. "Dr. Paterson will make it better soon." But Dr. Paterson had not made it better.

Yet, miraculously, Kevin continued to believe everything his mother said, and his trust made it necessary for her to believe everything she had told him.

She was on an emotional seesaw. One minute, she took on faith everything that Dr. Epstein told her. He seemed so friendly and real, with an underlying air of confidence that he could do the job. The next minute, she was vanquished by overwhelming doubt. Yet he continued to give her a feeling that the matter would be taken care of, just as he explained it.

Dr. Epstein had to know what he was talking about. After all, he'd been written up in the Reader's Digest and everyone said how good he was. Maybe it was silly, but she'd decided to check it out with JoAnn Baldwin, Fred's office manager.

"Do you have any children?" Ina Bea had asked her.

"Yes, a daughter," JoAnn had replied.

"If she had this . . . this problem, would you take her to Dr. Epstein?"

JoAnn put down the file and took both of Ina Bea's hands. "You mustn't worry," she said. "He's the best."

But just when Ina Bea thought she was convinced of that, dread took over, and she was back on the seesaw. Kevin had a brain tumor, he could die, no matter how good any doctor was or how comforting any doctor tried to be. Why did Dr. Epstein smile so much? All of a sudden, he seemed like a huckster, a snake-oil salesman pushing hope when there wasn't any.

It dawned on Ina Bea that she didn't know exactly how Dr. Epstein would get the tumor out. She envisioned a river of blood flowing from Kevin's head, like the one that had been there when he sliced his ear, and her knees started to buckle under her. She was going to call for a nurse when she felt someone take hold of her arm with a fierce grip. It was Carmen Olmedo, whose broad, strong face was full of concern.

Carmen held on to Ina Bea until the weakness passed. Then she moved a chair close to Kevin's bed.

"Siéntese aquí," she said.

"Thank you." For a moment, she was able to get out of herself, to empathize with Carmen, who was in a strange country, did not know the language, and had no one to help her. Ina Bea couldn't imagine going through this agony without Clay's love and support.

Kevin's voice interrupted her thoughts.

"Mom," he said, "do you remember when Dad and I were in the woods, and we saw that bear cub who was lost?"

"Yes."

"Well, that's how I feel, like a little cub bear. I'm lost in the woods and it's on fire, and I can't get out."

Ina Bea had to look away. She couldn't let him know that she felt just as lost.

All at once, a nurse was there giving Kevin some medication to make him sleepy, followed by an aide, a thin, young Hispanic man who tossed a greeting to Carmen Olmedo in Spanish. The aide lifted Kevin efficiently onto a gurney, then covered him with a blanket.

"We'll take good care of him, mommy," the young man said.

Ina Bea followed the gurney down the hall and watched it disappear into the elevator.

She sank down on one of the well-worn sofas by the elevator, on which so many parents had waited for news. The sofa was a typical piece of doctor's waiting room furniture. But where was the doctor, and what was he doing, and when oh when would he be finished?

She had her head in her hands when Clay appeared with a cup of coffee, a sweet roll, and a pile of magazines for her.

"They took Kevin down," Ina Bea said.

"Already?"

The news unsettled him.

"I said good-bye for you," Ina Bea lied. Clay had been the last thing on her mind.

Guiltily, she thumbed through her favorite women's magazine. A section of Thanksgiving recipies showed a picture of a dining room, the table groaning with holiday dishes and surrounded by plush Victorian side chairs, not unlike the Dagners' own.

"Nothing worth reading?"

She had been staring at the picture for how long—half an hour, an hour?

Clay moved closer and put his arm around her. What had he been thinking all this time? She was horrified to realize that she didn't care. Usually she was eager to share Clay's thoughts, to be a part of him, but now all she wanted was to be in her own private world—until Kevin came back to her safe again, or whatever way he would come back to her.

"Mind if I join you?" someone asked.

It was a young woman who had a blond ponytail and a shy smile. She appeared to be just out of her teens. At first, Ina Bea thought she was one of the patients, but then she learned that the woman's daughter, Barbie, was down on the operating floor, too, having a shunt replaced by one of Dr. Epstein's associates. A shunt, the young woman explained, was a device used to drain off excess fluid that sometimes accumulated in the head of a patient with a brain tumor.

Dr. Epstein had operated on Barbie's brainstem tumor three years ago, Jennifer Marting said, and put a shunt in beforehand to drain the cerebrospinal fluid. But fluid continued to back up afterward, and the shunt had become a permanent necessity. Barbie was, as the medical term went, "shunt dependent," and Jennifer had to be constantly alert to the possibility of a malfunction in the device.

"She got these real bad headaches, so I raced her down to Fred right away," Jennifer said, explaining that the family lived in New Jersey. "Where are you folks from?"

Clay took over the conversation and from time to time,

Ina Bea was aware of snatches of it. Barbie had recovered nicely, though at first, Jennifer said, she had worried about the shunt every single minute.

"I mean, it was like a time bomb. Whenever Barbie cried or even laughed very loud, I thought, 'This is it, she needs a replacement.' But then I calmed down. I mean, after a while, you get used to things."

Ina Bea's mind was racing. She hadn't thought about "after a while" and "getting used to things" or even about what would happen next. Dr. Epstein had told them only that Kevin would probably have to remain in the hospital about ten days and that he would be given medications.

But would Kevin have one of those shunt things in his head, and would it be there forever? It seemed horrible, but then a shiver came over her, and she chastised herself for worrying about a shunt when all that mattered was for Kevin to survive. Dr. Epstein had said there was a 7 percent chance that something might go wrong, paralysis or even worse. What if the worst was happening, right now, while she was sitting here?

Ina Bea stood up. "I'm going for a walk," she said.

"I'll go with you," Clay responded.

"No." She begged Clay to stay in the waiting area, in case there was some news.

She didn't know how she got out onto the street, but suddenly she was there, buttoning up her coat against the cold. Ina Bea had packed scarcely anything for herself, only this light raincoat and the print dress she was wearing. Yet she had brought along a full wardrobe for Kevin, pants and shirts and several changes of underwear, as if they were going on vacation.

I've been acting oddly, she thought, very oddly, but it didn't matter.

Soon she was on a busy shopping thoroughfare, with street vendors hawking their wares and signs on the store windows announcing GOING OUT OF BUSINESS sales, and everywhere more people than she had ever walked among before. They bumped against her, and the random contact numbed Ina Bea and helped her stop thinking so much about the operation.

She walked on with absolutely no idea of what she was looking at or whose path she was blocking, her thoughts going back to the day of Kevin's birth. It was Clay who had done the walking then, all over town, he said, and back again, several times, till everyone knew that Ina Bea was in the community hospital, at last having the child she had wanted for so long.

She remembered the hospital smells, so similar to those of New York University Medical Center, and how Kevin had looked when they handed him to her wrapped in a blanket, and she'd thought, "I'm going to take good care of you," just the words the orderly had used this morning.

Suddenly Ina Bea realized that she had no idea where she was, but somehow she managed to find a taxicab.

The driver, perhaps alarmed by her pallor and her an-nounced destination, asked what was wrong. Ina Bea told him, in a weak voice, that her son was being operated on, right this very minute, for a brain tumor.

When they arrived at the hospital and she started to fumble through her purse, the driver told her to forget about the fare.

"Just hurry up inside," he said.

She flew into Clay's arms, really looking at him, it seemed, for the first time that day.

"Any news?" she asked.

"Not yet, but Tania's been here several times and sat with me for a while. She says she's been in the OR and everything is going just as it should."

"It seems to be taking so long," Ina Bea commented.

Clay smiled. "Tania told me every parent feels that way."

Their hours of waiting finally came to a close. The operation ended and Kevin was brought to the recovery room. He was in the capable hands of Murray Canter, who bent over him, his salt-and-pepper beard almost touching the boy's face.

"Can you hear me, Kevin?" Murray boomed. He had begun to reverse the anesthetic, even before they left OR, and he removed the breathing tube as soon as Kevin demonstrated the capacity to breathe on his own. Little by little, Kevin was freed of the leads and wires that had been affixed to him for nearly six hours. Only the IV remained, supplying fluids to prevent dehydration, and a drainage tube had been inserted in the wound.

Kevin nodded sleepily, then opened his eyes and smiled.

"Everything's okay," Mike Wilson said. "You'll see your parents in a little while."

Mike elevated Kevin's head—the way it would remain from now on—and performed a neurological examination, checking the boy's pupils and testing his reflexes.

"Don't go to sleep on me now, Kevin," Mike pleaded.

He tugged gently at his arm, and Kevin returned to consciousness.

"Now we're going to play a game, 'this little piggy,' remember that one?" Mike said. "Show me how you can move your toes, the big one and all of them."

Kevin shook his head weakly and drifted off again. Was he only sleepy or was something terribly wrong?

"Kevin," Murray urged, "Come on, old pal. You're an athlete. It's the big game. Move those toes."

He and Mike stared at Kevin's right foot. One husky toe began to wriggle and then the others.

Murray breathed an audible sigh of relief.

"Tell Fred he can talk with the parents now," he said to Mike.

When Fred found the Dagners, he was still wearing his scrubs and green clogs.

"Everything's fine," he said, seating himself and looking directly into Ina Bea's eyes. "Kevin's going to be okay. I got most of the tumor."

"Oh, Dr. Epstein, I'm so glad," Ina Bea said. She began to smile, but then the floodgates opened and tears streamed down her face.

Fred reached out and put his hand on her shoulder, and he could feel some of the tension go out of her. He knew what her morning had been like, waves of anxiety and terror accompanied by undercurrents of hope and doubt. Some parents sat silently, some went to the chapel to pray, some fidgeted and talked with everyone in sight, some left the hospital and prowled the streets, some snapped at the staff nurses or at Tania. Be patient, Fred told his staff; put yourself in the parents' situation.

Now, he knew, the Dagners were basking in the golden peace of relief, but that would soon be followed by new concerns and questions as they realized that Kevin's life—and theirs—had been changed forever.

"You said 'most' of the tumor. Does that mean it could come back?" Clay asked.

"It might, but I'm hopeful that it won't. My concern is not about the immediate future, but what'll happen down the line," Fred replied.

Ina Bea remembered Clay's talk with Jennifer Marting.

"Dr. Epstein, will Kevin need to have something in his head to drain the fluid?" she asked.

"A shunt? No, I don't think so," Fred replied, "not if we're able to control the swelling. Usually children who need shunts had a great deal of swelling before the operation, and Kevin didn't."

Clay Dagner cut in with his questions. When would Kevin be able to talk? To run? Would he be able to play sports again? And what about his schoolwork? Would his mind be okay? Would he still have pain?

"Don't jump six steps ahead," Fred said softly. "You'll drive yourself crazy. From now on, we're going to take this each day at a time."

They hung on his every word, and he realized that he was speaking a new gospel, one that they would repeat to themselves over and over again. "Take it easy, Ina Bea, remember what Dr. Epstein said, 'Don't jump six steps ahead.' " There was a long future ahead, he hoped, for Kevin Dagner, but not one, unfortunately, that would be free of worry.

He reassured the Dagners that kids were very resilient and recovered more quickly than adults from brain surgery. They were also better at fighting back from any problems that might develop.

Fred took hold of Ina Bea's plump hands. "Look," he said. "We're holding on together. We want the same results in this war. And we're going to win."

Ina Bea saw how deeply Fred felt about Kevin, and his energy began to buoy her up, coming as it seemed to from an inexhaustible source. She could see that he took Kevin's illness as a personal challenge, almost as if her son were a member of his own family. Ina Bea also sensed his strong need to be liked, just as she, right now, needed someone to like her.

All at once, it felt as though she had known this Dr. Epstein all her life.

"You can see Kevin now," he said, telling the Dagners how to reach the recovery room. "We'll talk later, whenever you want. My door is always open."

There was a squeeze and a hug for Ina Bea, while Clay Dagner looked on.

Then Clay shook the doctor's hand solemnly. "Thank you . . . Fred." It was the first time that either of the Dagners had called him by his given name. Their real relationship had begun.

A few moments later, Fred was in a room down the hall.

The patient, a thirteen-year-old black girl, sat at the foot of her bed looking like a giant doll with round brown eyes, a round, smooth face, and a bevy of braids falling from her head in an asymmetrical pattern.

"Are you all ready for tomorrow, Leslie?" Fred asked, gently forcing her head downward so that he could feel the traces of an old scar. This was a recurrence, Leslie having been operated on by another surgeon in another hospital several years previously.

"Hey, I'm afraid we're going to have to spoil that hairdo," Fred said.

"I told her not to get it done like that," Mrs. Frazier said, with a blend of exasperation and fear in her voice. She leaned against the wall, a carbon copy of her daughter, wearing a tight T-shirt and jeans. At the foot of Leslie's bed, her teenage brother sat. He had an earring in one ear and a scowl on his face, apparently having decided, like many teenagers, to display bravado rather than concern.

"Is Leslie gonna get better this time?" he asked.

"You bet," Fred said firmly.

The boy looked him up and down and finally relaxed his facial muscles a bit.

I hope he really cares about her, Fred thought; she's going to need him now.

Fred asked Mrs. Frazier if she had any questions, and heard

the usual: "How long will it take?" "Where should we meet you?"

"Don't be concerned about the hair, Leslie," Fred said. "We'll manage, and we'll shave as little as possible, I promise."

"Do whatever you have to. Just do it right," the girl replied, with an intensity that made it clear she wasn't only talking about her hair. Then she turned her glance away from him.

Fred recoiled slightly and chewed at the inside of his lower lip.

"Don't worry, Leslie," he said, patting her on the shoulder. "I'll take care of you."

He wasn't out of the room two minutes before he began to think about the operating plan.

CHAPTER 10

FRED

I left the hospital shortly after dusk, hoping to surprise Kathy by getting home at a reasonable hour, but I ran into a traffic jam on the East River Drive. When I saw flashing lights far up ahead of me, signaling either an accident or a construction tie-up, I realized I was in for a long wait.

Bad news, because I get antsy if I'm stuck in one place. Perhaps it has something to do with my long legs or my short attention span, but whatever it is, I have to be up and moving. I can sit and think about a problem for only so long—not very long, my co-workers say—and then I have to do something about it and move on to the next thing.

Though I take lots of time to talk with parents and patients, I'm never totally relaxed. In fact, Tania says restlessness sticks to me the same way dirt sticks to Pigpen, the character in the "Peanuts" comic strip.

A neurosurgery practice is stressful, and Tania relieves the tension by using relaxation techniques, but they don't work for me. To relax, I have to be physically away from the hospital, at my vacation home on Fire Island, for example. Even on summer weekends out there, though, I'm only relaxed on Friday. By Saturday, I'm stalking again, moving from place to place in search of something to do. The exception is when I'm out on my sailboat, where I can remain happily for hours.

I've been sailing since I was a child, and there's something about being alone on the water that's totally soothing. Sailing is one of the things I did best when I was young, and I sometimes wonder if it didn't set my future course for surgery. Like a sailor, a neurosurgeon is basically alone, in control, and dependent on his or her ability to take risks, a fairly good description of me.

Just thinking about the open sea made me feel better, but I was very far from it now. Trapped like a rat and hungry, too. I looked around the car for traces of the snack foods I love so much, but the only edible I found was a container of diet drink, which I had hidden from Kathy. I sipped at it guiltily, knowing how much she wants me to eat balanced meals rather than alternating, as I often do, between fast food and diet stuff.

"What did you have for lunch?" she'll ask me. I always claim I don't remember, but the fact is that, on the run, I may have had pizza, Chinese food, homemade fudge, or perhaps all three, depending on how much JoAnn ordered out or what goodies a patient's parent gave us. My staff and I don't get out for lunch very often, so snacking and ordering out are passions. More than hunger is involved, I'm sure. The fact is, the food shores us up emotionally and gets our minds off a lot of worry and sadness.

As I sipped the diet drink, I thought about Kevin Dagner's surgery, which had gone quite well. The report from the intensive care unit had been encouraging, too. Kevin's vital signs were good, his intracranial pressure was within expected bounds of elevation, and he wasn't complaining very much about post-op pain. In fact, he said, he felt "pretty okay" because the severe pain caused by the tumor was gone.

So I'd been justified in giving the Dagners a positive report. But a lot could happen in the next few days. I'd seen kids wake up fine in the recovery room and then, later on, develop some dysfunction: problems in breathing and swallowing, a dangerous increase in intracranial pressure, infection, or seizures, since surgery temporarily disturbs the normal function of brain cells.

It's always a struggle to decide exactly how much to tell parents about what might happen. Say too much and they become overwhelmed; say too little and they're unprepared if things go wrong.

Perhaps I'm too upbeat, but over the years, I've found that it's best to err on the side of optimism. Maybe it's because I desperately need to feel optimistic myself. It tears me up when things go badly, when a patient needs a tracheostomy tube to breathe, for example. But would it have helped his parents if I'd warned them in advance? I doubt it.

Over the years, I've concluded that it's best to discuss a problem when it happens, rather than anticipate it. Because you can never say for certain what will happen. Kids simply don't follow the rules. Some are alive five years after you thought they'd be dead, and some who seem to be doing great die rather quickly.

No one knows what lies ahead except that even the best recovery will be rocky. Tania tells parents that they have to learn to pace themselves, like marathon runners, and I do the same, giving out information in increments.

"Let's talk later," I'd said to the Dagners before they went off to see Kevin in the recovery room. I'd need to prepare them for the way Kevin would look in a few days as the steroids, prescribed to relieve intracranial pressure, made his face look puffy or swollen.

Later on, the Dagners would learn that Kevin needed physical therapy and that there might be residual problems, such as a weakness on one side of his body. There could be learning problems, too.

Nonetheless, I had a feeling that things would go well with Kevin, and that he'd be able to resume a normal life. If that happened, he would owe his survival not to me, but to high technology, like the MRI, and new instrumentation, such as that ultrasonic marvel, the Cavitron.

When I was being trained, we were taught that most brain-stem tumors were inoperable; one reason was that we had no map to locate them specifically and learn their size. In 1985, nuclear magnetic resonance imaging, now known as MRI, changed that. Not only is MRI noninvasive, as no contrast agents are required, but it also clearly delineates the tumor's size and location.

Also, before the Cavitron was developed for brain surgery at New York University Medical Center in the 1970s, there was no safe way to excise brainstem tumors. Conventional instruments put too much pressure on normal tissues to risk using them in a region that controlled breathing and other vital bodily functions.

By contrast, in expert hands the Cavitron exerted no pressure at all, since the vibrating tip fragmented even the firmest tissues and simultaneously removed the residue by suction. In that function it was similar to its namesake, the Cavitron dental scaler, which had been used by dentists since the mid-fifties to remove plaque and to suck up blood and tartar. Later, ophthalmologists would alter the equipment and use it to remove cataracts.

In the early 1970s, Joe Ransohoff and other neurosurgeons at NYU began research with animal studies, trying to adapt the Cavitron's unique properties for brain surgery. It was risky, but exciting, challenging, on the edge. The way I like it.

I watched their work with fascination, learning the technique. There was no doubt that it permitted us to do surgery more quickly and with less trauma to adjacent tissues.

I started using the Cavitron on children in the late 1970s. Many of my early cases were desperate and seemingly hopeless. Some of the patients had been treated with heavy doses of radiation followed by chemotherapy, and been sent home to die. The Cavitron, along with the operating microscope and other innovative instruments, offered them their first real chance of getting better.

One of my earliest cases, Roger Hendricks, on whom I operated in 1980, reminded me a great deal of Kevin Dagner, and his parents were strong, down-to-earth people like Ina Bea and Clay.

The Hendrickses lived in a town in the Midwest. One day, when Roger was four, he began to scream, tightly clutching his head. The Hendrickses assumed that he'd been stung by a bee, but two weeks later, the same thing happened.

The emergency room physician thought the pain might have something to do with the fact that Roger's ear canal was "shaped differently." The pediatrician ordered a CT (computed tomography) scan—this was before we had MRIs—but nothing showed up. Like the Dagner's doctor, he concluded that the patient was suffering from an obscure form of migraine headache but that it was, as he wrote in the medical record, "nothing terminal." He couldn't have been more wrong.

The Hendrickses suffered for a year with screaming episodes of unbelievable intensity. Little Roger would clutch his head and flail about on the sofa, yelling like a person being burned in a fire. He ripped out his hair. Once he screamed for thirty-two hours straight.

The tumor was finally diagnosed when Roger suffered a stroke, and the local hospital sent him by ambulance to a larger hospital in a nearby city.

"Is he going to die?" Mr. Hendricks asked the physician there.

"With radiation to reduce the size of the tumor, he has six months to a year."

The radiation treatment began around Roger's fifth birthday and went on for six weeks. Even so, he had no relief from the pain. Roger grabbed at his chest so fiercely that he actually tore a hole in it, straight through the cartilage.

After radiation, there was chemotherapy, which produced some additional shrinkage of the tumor, but no cessation of the pain.

All the time this was going on, Mrs. Hendricks asked repeatedly, "Isn't there someone, somewhere, who can cure Roger?"

Nobody had the answer, though our work with the Cavitron had already received some attention. Even today, it's not well known in many parts of the United States that certain brain-stem tumors are operable, and parents are often told to take a child home to die when something could have been done. That's why it's imperative for parents with a seriously ill child to go to a major medical center, where the latest information is disseminated.

Fortunately for the Hendrickses, a physician who knew me heard about the case and referred them to me. They flew in at once, and I met with them in my office at midnight.

"There are five possibilities," I told them. "Roger could die during surgery, lapse into a coma, become paralyzed, wind up no worse off than he was before, or get better." I figured the chances of the latter happening at 20 percent because of the extent and duration of the tumor, and also because we didn't have enough statistics on the success of the Cavitron to offer a better percentage.

Mrs. Hendricks didn't think about what I had said for more than a second. She and her husband were born-again Christians, she told me.

"Two weeks ago," she went on, "the Lord told me that He would heal Roger. I want you to operate, Dr. Epstein."

The surgery had to be delayed for some weeks because the chemotherapeutic drugs had suppressed Roger's white blood cell production, and his weight was down sharply.

While we waited, Roger, now six years old, received volumes of narcotics and sedatives, and yet his pain continued. Part of it was mental. He flinched in terror every time he saw anyone wearing white—I took off my white coat whenever I examined him—or anything that looked remotely like a medical instrument. He had been tortured by physicians almost as much as he had been by the tumor. I had never seen a child in so much pain.

The morning of the surgery, Roger was hysterical with fear, crying that he didn't want to go to the operating room. I was worried about the effect of his emotional state on the surgery, so I asked the anesthesiologist to put him to sleep in his room.

"It's not safe, Fred," the doctor said with deep concern. "He's very fragile. He could go into shock, have respiratory failure, anything. I'd be helpless here. All my equipment's in the OR."

"Do it, please," I insisted. "I'll take responsibility."

Roger's arm was so emaciated that it was difficult to find a vein, but after several tries, we finally inserted an IV and began an infusion of sodium pentothal.

I cradled the boy in my arms and, even though he was anesthetized, I talked to him all the way down to the sixth floor. "You're going to be fine, Roger. Soon it won't hurt anymore." I could have sworn that he heard me.

Roger's tumor was intramedullary, located within the upper part of the spinal cord and the lower area of the brainstem called the medulla. When we opened, I could see the tumor immediately; it was bulging and causing the entire region to look swollen and distorted.

I began to resect—or remove—the tumor, using the Cavitron. When I reached the area between the first and third cervical nerves, the anesthesiologist asked me to stop for a moment.

"He's having a lot of pain, Fred, and I mean a lot."

The monitors showed pronounced tachycardia, increased heartbeat, which could have resulted from the irritation of pain-sensitive tissue.

It was incredible. Roger was deeply anesthetized, and he'd been loaded down with narcotics for months, even years, yet the pain caused by that damn tumor continued. There was no choice, though, but to go on, which I did with increased awareness of the fragile little being beneath the sterile drapes.

As I approached the obex, the junction of a band of fibers at the fourth ventricle of the brain, Roger developed bradycardia, a slowed-down heartbeat. I was afraid his heart would stop.

"Talk to me," I said to the anesthesiologist. I needed to know if he had administered any drugs that might have altered the heartbeat. But the bradycardia was not drug-induced—a clear signal that it was no longer possible to pursue the tumor safely.

I wasn't sure how much of the tumor I'd gotten out. I estimated it at about 70 percent, less than I would have liked, but the pathology report confirmed that the tumor was benign, as I had suspected it would be. Often, if I remove a large piece of a benign tumor, the part left behind can wither. I was hopeful that would be the case here.

When he regained consciousness, Roger was more free of pain than he had been in years. He twitched a bit, and his parents worried that he might be having a seizure, but I explained that the twitching was caused by withdrawal from the vast number of drugs he had been on.

For the first few weeks post-op, the left side of Roger's body was weak, almost paralyzed. He went home that way. But by the time I saw him six months later, his body had become much stronger and he was able to stop using the wheelchair he had been confined to. He was also able to attend school for the first time in his life.

Roger needed a program of physical therapy to improve his strength, balance, and coordination, and speech therapy to improve the clarity of his speech. He continued with these therapies for years, but they paid off.

Today, Roger Hendricks is seventeen years old, plays baseball, rides a bicycle, and makes outstanding grades in school. He no longer flinches when he sees a medical professional. In fact, he's less scared of life than many young people his age who have never been sick a day in their lives.

That isn't to say there aren't problems. Roger still has

recurrent episodes of facial pain, some trouble swallowing, and he tends to hold his head to the left side. His early CT scans showed that there was no tumor left, but the more recent MRI scans, which give us a better picture than the CT, show that something is still there. I'm confident, however, that what we see is the withered remainder of the tumor.

I can imagine what his parents must go through every time a scan looks "strange." "This stuff blows your mind," one mother told me after such an incident. Still, worry is part of the legacy of having survived a brain tumor, actually part of the good news.

I think of all the parents I know who'd be glad to endure this anxiety if only their child were still alive; God knows what I'd be willing to endure if only I could have saved their child.

When I'm alone, as I was now in my car, memories of patients who have died come back to me, and I begin to run tapes of them through my mind. I'm not good at names—abysmal, in fact—but I can remember every one of theirs.

I prayed that Kevin Dagner's name wouldn't be one I'd think about on some dark night in some other lonely place.

I prayed for Luis Olmedo, too, and I was considerably more worried about him. Luis's spinal cord astrocytoma was malignant, which made the prognosis much more ominous.

Four years ago, I had gone to the funeral of another patient, who had had a similar tumor. Frank Morella, Jr., was a high school sophomore with everything going for him: varsity football team, honor society, lots of friends and most important, a fine and loving nature.

His symptoms came on suddenly—sharp back pain and increasing weakness, resulting in paralysis within two months.

Frank started the football season as a quarterback, but by the time the season was half over, he was on the sidelines, in a wheelchair.

I performed a laminotomy, a surgical procedure that removes the vertebrae so the dura is visible. Carefully, I opened the dura; then with the laser, I did a myelotomy, an incision to open the spinal cord. Using the Cavitron, I removed 95 percent of the tumor. Because Frank's symptoms had come on so rapidly, a characteristic of malignancy, I feared the worst.

"Astrocytoma, Grade III," confirmed the pathology report.

When I told the news to Frank Morella, Sr., a big, husky construction worker, he broke down and wept, making agonized noises that scarcely seemed to be human.

But a few minutes later, when he spoke to his son, he was calm and matter-of-fact.

"We're going to do everything we can, Frankie," he said, holding his once-strong son close and looking at me as if he had given me marching orders.

I wasn't quite sure then that there would be an "everything." At the time, we had very little experience with this rare type of tumor, having treated only eight other cases, none with great success.

Some people might have thought there was a case for doing nothing, but that wasn't my opinion. It wasn't as if Frank would have died in peace if I'd left him alone. Quite the contrary, the pain caused by the growing tumor would have given him greater discomfort than any procedure I could devise.

The other reason to be aggressive was that we might be successful. Sarah Glazer had proven to me over and over again the unpredictability of cancer. The will to live cannot be overestimated and neither can the importance of hope.

"Nothing is too wonderful to be true," Michael Faraday, the nineteenth-century physicist, once said. Perhaps Frank's tumor would not recur if we did "everything."

In following the wishes of Frank Senior, I would also be following my own.

Frank was given a tremendous dose of radiation, four thousand rads, followed by chemotherapy, and for a short time, he seemed to be making progress.

Then our hopes were dashed. Six months after the first operation, Frank was suddenly unable to move his arms. A second surgery offered the only hope, and a slim one at that, of preventing total paralysis.

I didn't even wait to learn what the myelogram—an X ray in which a radiopaque dye is injected into the subarachnoid space in order to allow one to visualize the spinal cord—would show about the extent of the tumor; I rushed Frank to the OR. In spite of my efforts, he emerged from the operation a quadriplegic.

Frank blamed no one, not me, not life, not fate. He'd talk about his friends and what was happening at the high school, and he'd tease his sister. He was in pain, and he was sad, but he had the most incredible inner strength. He refused to give up. The more his health declined, the more he seemed to be supporting his family spiritually. He wanted to live, and they wanted him to be alive. We decided to go on fighting.

Frank was placed on a protocol of carboplatinum, an extremely powerful drug that was being studied at the time and has since proved to be effective with some types of brain and spinal tumors.

The drug provided a short gift of time, one last Christmas. As a present, Frank gave his parents a picture he had painted by holding a brush in his teeth.

A few weeks later, he developed hydrocephalus because the tumor had metastasized to his brain. A shunt was put in to relieve the pressure and after that, I wrote in my notes, "no further treatment is anticipated."

When I told him that the fight had ended, Mr. Morella put his hand over his eyes, but he didn't cry.

The waiting began and the watching as Frank's body failed, system after system. His mother described it as "waiting for the next horror, for something else to break down."

Within a short while, Frank fell into a coma. His parents took turns staying with their son until he died.

Frank was truly one of God's best efforts, and I value everything that was done to try to save him. Even if chances for survival are slim, parents are usually comforted by the knowledge that they did their best, and the battle itself can affirm their love for the child.

"We were all blessed by Frankie," Mr. Morella told me at the funeral. "Being his father was a privilege, and I would gladly accept the suffering we went through again, because he was worth it."

Undoubtedly, Carmen Olmedo also thought that Luis was worth everything; so why had she come to the decision she made? I felt I had failed to convey the situation to her with a sense of hope, probably because of the language barrier. The word "optimism" can be translated, but how to translate the feeling of optimism, a feeling that can sustain and perhaps even cure?

All of a sudden, I saw that I'd given Carmen too many medical facts and too little of myself. Weighed down by translation problems and a passion to operate, I'd broken my own rule, the one I'd written about in an article for pediatric neurosurgeons: "Our obligations transcend the mechanical performance of even a complex surgical procedure and include a commitment to become part of a distraught family in its moment of need."

I resolved to work my way into Carmen's life somehow, to understand what she was thinking. The Olmedos had four other children and a grandmother living with them. Maybe their economic resources, already pitiful, had deteriorated. Maybe Carmen had had to go to work. Maybe the grandmother wasn't capable of caring for a sick child and four well children. What other maybes had I overlooked?

A horn honked behind me, and I realized that cars up ahead were moving. I inched along, the comparative burst of freedom banishing all thoughts but my desire to get home.

Kathy and the kids were still seated around the dinner table, finishing dessert. Jason, our oldest son, was recounting one of his matches from the recent wrestling season.

"Dad, remember when the coach bumped me up to the 130-pound-weight class even though I was five pounds under?" he asked.

"Sure do," I replied.

A big smile spread over his face, the kind of smile that makes you want to hug a kid, whether he's talking about a match or how much better he feels after an operation.

"I pinned that guy. Outmaneuvered him completely." Then Jason's smile vanished rather too quickly. "Still, we lost the tournament," he said, recalling the meet's sad conclusion.

"Well, there's always the next time," I assured him.

There I was again, the eternal optimist.

Even as a young boy, I thought things would work out, especially if I made an effort. "You really believe you can make a difference, don't you, Fred?" my father would ask when I suggested some scheme or other.

In a way, my optimism was ironic, because in school I had little reason to feel hopeful about things. It was sheer torture, day after day, to have to look at letters and numbers that didn't make any sense and to realize that yet another crummy report card was going to be sent home.

My father was endlessly kind, but I didn't know how much faith he had in my ability to learn. It was my aunt Lottie, my mother's sister, who fanned my optimism. She lived near the school I attended and, having some time on her hands, resolved to help me with my writing.

I remember long hours spent at her dining room table, listening to her soothing voice: "Think about what you're trying to say, Fred. What point do you want to make?" Hour after hour, she never seemed to lose her patience. If a session went badly, she'd say, "Tomorrow is another day."

It was indeed. And though I still don't find writing easy, I've published more than 140 medical articles to date. Too bad Aunt Lottie didn't live to read them. She would have enjoyed reading them, I'm sure, even if she had only the foggiest idea of what they were about.

The telephone rang, and Kathy answered it.

"It's Lila Glazer," she said, her slim hand over the phone.

I knew Lila wouldn't bother me at home unless she was very worried. What could have happened between this call and the time I'd seen her and Daniel at the hospital, a little over an hour ago?

"Fred, I'm calling from the nurses' station. I left Daniel in Sarah's room," Lila whispered. "I'm so scared, and it's not only that she's dying. It's that Daniel just won't accept what's happening."

"I know," I said.

"I never thought I'd see him like this, never. He just started talking about how we'll be taking Sarah home soon. And he accused me of losing hope. Hope? Fred, you know what she looks like, but Daniel doesn't seem to see. I'm so worried about him."

I was worried, too.

There's a thin line between knowing when to fight for a child and when to surrender, almost like the imperceptible change in color between the edges of a tumor and normal tissue, but most parents seem to recognize the line instinctively. Then they start to make agonizing emotional adjustments.

Lila was in the midst of that adjustment process now, but Daniel, who had seen the battle lost and then won again so often, refused to join her, thereby increasing everyone's pain, including Sarah's.

Children of Sarah's age know when they're dying, and when adults refuse to help them say good-bye, the leave-taking becomes even more difficult. Sometimes they feel they have to hang on to accommodate a parent's wishes, when every inch of their diseased bodies aches for rest.

"Fred, can't you do something?" Lila said.

I could hear the weariness in her voice. How long had it been since she had a good night's sleep or had been able to spend any time with her other child, Naomi?

"Tell Daniel I'll be right there," I said.

CHAPTER 11

A few hours later, Daniel Glazer sat in the study of his suburban home, still moved by Fred's having hurried back to the hospital to talk with him.

At first glance, the study could have belonged to any rabbi. On the desk, there was a pile of letters from congregants and colleagues, a calendar of synagogue events, and future sermons in various stages of completion. Certificates on the wall attested to Daniel's ordination, advanced degrees, and the congregation's successful participation in a recent fund-raising endeavor. The bookcases held volumes on theology and history and several dog-eared commentaries on Jewish law.

Only one bookcase was different. It contained textbooks on neurology and neurosurgery and a pile of articles on brain tumors, most of them written by Fred J. Epstein, M.D. Daniel, in his endless quest for mastery, had pored over almost all of Fred's writings, even those that had nothing to do with problems like Sarah's.

"When will you be scrubbing up?" Fred had joked during one of his visits to the Glazers' suburban New Jersey home.

Daniel laughed, but in truth he would have liked to go into the OR, to have been capable of saving his daughter's life himself. One of the frustrating aspects of Sarah's illness was the constant sense of helplessness. A parent should be able to protect his child, but the tumor had stripped that power from him. Never had helplessness gripped Daniel more completely than it did this night, as he sat in the study thinking about his conversation with Fred earlier in the evening.

"You've done everything you can do for Sarah," Fred had said. "Now you may have to do the hardest thing of all—help her to die."

Daniel almost fainted at the words. All of these years, ever since Sarah's first miraculous remission, it had been Fred's optimism that kept Daniel going. Sometimes he could feel it in his legs and arms, actually holding him up when he wanted to lie down on the ground and never move again.

Now Fred, the familiar harbinger of hope, had suddenly turned into the bearer of a terrible truth.

Stormy memories raged over Daniel as he looked out the window into the pitiless night.

It was in this very room that Sarah first became ill when she was six months old. Daniel was giving her the early evening feeding, when suddenly she pushed the bottle out of her mouth. A second later, she was having convulsions, her head, neck, and arms shaking with spasms. Then she lost consciousness.

A few hours later, a Dr. Epstein, whom they didn't know, was "exploring" Sarah's brain. The Glazers met Fred at four o'clock in the morning when he came from the OR. There was nothing to be done, he told them, as direct as a surgical knife, yet the room seemed to explode with sympathetic energy, the energy of Fred sharing himself.

"I know it's hell," he said, his eyebrows moving up and down intently. "It's unimaginable," as if the unimaginable were happening to him.

There was some discussion, Daniel remembered, about radiation. Fred advised against it, saying that even if the treatment reduced the tumor, it could be harmful to the healthy part of the infant's brain.

"Radiation isn't for very young children," Fred explained, but he referred them to a neurooncologist for a consultation just the same.

"You'll be derelict in your duty if you don't have the radiation," the specialist told them.

The Glazers were torn, recognizing for the first time that they had entered an area with conflicting answers to each of their questions.

They decided to do as Fred advised and took Sarah home to die. But she didn't die. Over the next three years, she surprised them all by developing normally. She was talking at a year, walking a short time later, and showed no evidence of brain damage.

"Thank you, God," Daniel prayed as CT scans showed that the tumor was shrinking without treatment.

"What do you make of it?" he asked Fred.

"Frankly, I'm shocked," Fred replied. "Really flabbergasted. It's very rare for this to happen. In fact, I've never seen it with this type of a tumor."

That should have been a warning, but Daniel took it as a confirmation that the miracle would continue. When the tumor started to hemorrhage a few months short of Sarah's fourth birthday, he was devastated.

But Fred's optimism, after he operated to stop the bleeding, gave Daniel hope.

"She's old enough for our fight for her to begin in earnest," Fred had informed the Glazers. "There are things we can do now we couldn't do before."

Daniel would never forget that first course of radiation and chemotherapy, with Sarah fatigued and complaining of upset stomachs, but mostly concerned about her loss of hair.

"I'm not bootiful anymore," she said with a four-year-old lisp, perched on the bathroom sink and looking in the mirror.

"Of course you are," Daniel said, hugging her close. He realized that they would have to fight the effects of the illness on her self-image as well as on her body, another front in this seemingly endless war.

Lila, having quit her job, spent every waking minute with Sarah. They let the housekeeper go and with only one income, had to sell their spacious Colonial home and move into a modest ranch.

"What good would a beautiful house be without Sarah in it?" Lila asked as she sorted through the possessions they would be giving away in the move.

Sarah's illness honed both of them down to the spiritual bone, Lila's materialism evaporating along with Daniel's easy, optimistic faith. They became a couple who judged the universe by posing one question—Why did things like this happen to small children?—and daily life against one measure—How would this or that decision affect Sarah?

There was a forgotten figure in all of this, their first child, Naomi, Sarah's senior by three years.

One night, when Sarah was particularly ill with the side effects of chemo treatment, seven-year-old Naomi crawled up on Daniel's knee.

"Did I do it?" she asked as he stroked her hair.

"Do what, honey?"

"The tumor, Daddy," Naomi replied, her voice shaking. "Remember, you said I used to poke Sarah when she was just born."

"Of course not, Naomi. No one caused the tumor. It was just something that happened." Those were Fred's words, and Daniel had to believe them.

What else was Naomi thinking?

"It's not catching, either," Daniel went on, and he could feel her small body relax. "And you know what—you can even go right on poking Sarah, but not all the time."

They both laughed, and Daniel thought he had won on another front, the struggle to preserve an air of normalcy.

"These illnesses are very hard on siblings," Fred confirmed when Daniel told him the story. "They blame themselves or they get angry at being left out of the patient's care."

"I won't leave her out," Daniel vowed.

A year later, Sarah hemorrhaged again, and Fred performed another craniotomy. This time, the convalescence was complicated by a bout of meningitis and when it was over, Sarah, pale and wasted, was more precious to them than ever.

Lila refused to have any nurses at home, handling everything herself with the able assistance of Naomi, who took pride in giving Sarah her medications.

"You've got to spell yourself," Tania said. "Hire some help or ask a friend to come in." Lila refused. "If I let go of Sarah, she will die," she insisted.

Even Daniel felt pushed out of the way, but Lila's efforts paid off. Sarah got better, and the memory of her lying in the hospital, her face bloated beyond recognition by steroids, faded from their minds.

At six, Sarah was enthusiastic, loving, and cute—her hair had grown back in little corkscrew curls—but she was highly distractible. She couldn't sit still while Daniel read her a story and rarely finished a game with her sister.

Lila volunteered at the preschool Sarah attended until Sarah "graduated," and the Glazers learned that the local public school had no program for special-education youngsters.

"I'm going to start a school," Lila said.

She convinced the synagogue to donate space, and she wrote a grant proposal to an education foundation. Within six months, there was a "school," with twenty-eight students, four teachers, and a board of directors, headed by Lila.

Those were good years. Daniel remembered Sarah learning to read and write and take part in plays and athletic events, even though her speech was slurred and her gait unsteady. Each small achievement was a triumph. When she managed to jump rope, with himself and Lila turning the rope slowly, Daniel was delirious with joy and a sense of good fortune.

"You have to live for the moment," Fred said, whenever Daniel asked him how long that fortune would continue. Daniel learned to judge happiness by a different standard, treasuring each day that was pain free or showed progress.

With Fred, the Glazers shared photographs, drawings, and Sarah's single-paragraph "compositions." They all went into a special "Sarah" file, Fred commented, right behind her medical files.

All too soon, it seemed, those medical records grew more voluminous as Sarah experienced a series of setbacks. There were other hemorrhages, craniotomies to control them, and, once, an abscess in the space where the tumor had been.

Each time, Lila said to Fred: "I want you to fix it," and he tried.

The abscess had permanently damaged a section of bone, which had to be removed and the opening repaired by a plastic surgeon. The procedure took eight hours, and then the insurance company refused to pay for what it considered a "cosmetic" operation.

Lila cried when she got the form letter. "It's the last goddamned straw," she told Fred.

Fred put Rochelle Sedita, his office assistant who handled insurance claims, on the case. The two of them badgered the company until it paid up.

"A plastic surgeon is utilized in this type of operation because it is very difficult to close a wound of this kind. An area that has been previously operated on needs a very tight closure so that you will not have leakage of cerebrospinal fluid," Fred wrote.

He didn't say that self-image was crucial to a child's unique ability to compensate for neurological defects. The repair work was scarcely visible. Sarah was still "bootiful."

She returned to school and the Glazers to their pretense of normalcy, but Sarah knew she was different.

"I have a tumor," she wrote in one composition, "and radiation isn't that great."

Sometimes Sarah used the tumor as a tool with which to manipulate her family. If Naomi teased her, she would say in slurred tones, "Stop it, or I'll have a tumor attack." Once she complained that the tumor made it hard for her to complete an assigned task of sweeping the kitchen floor.

"No such luck, young lady," Daniel said, putting the broom back into her shaky hand. Then he watched her sweep the small area, a job that took her twenty minutes. A normal child would have done it in a flash, but Daniel no longer thought about normalcy. He only thought about the glow on Sarah's face when she got finished and how he swept her up in his arms and kissed her—another moment to be treasured.

Concentrating on Sarah, grabbing what time he could with Naomi, Daniel at first failed to realize how exhausted Lila had become. Maybe it was because she refused to acknowledge it herself.

When she wasn't at the school, or taking Sarah to the physical therapist or the speech therapist, she was thinking about things that could be done for other Sarahs, ways in which the health-care system could be reformed.

"You've got to slow down," Daniel said one night, looking at Lila's haggard face.

"What do you know about it?" she shot back. "You're not here all day."

It wasn't fair. He tried to be there as much as possible, but someone had to support the family and take care of a clergyman's myriad responsibilities.

Members of the congregation volunteered to relieve Lila, and increasingly she let them. But she quickly grew impatient, claiming that they didn't know how to do this or that. She was really frightened, Daniel realized, that something terrible might happen while she was gone.

Still, she agreed to get out of the house more, provided that she wore a beeper at her waist. When Daniel commented that the beeper contravened the purpose of having a peaceful time away, she shook her head.

"I have to be in touch," she insisted.

And in touch she was, through a never-ending cycle of good and bad.

Daniel could no longer remember when this craniotomy had occurred, or that infection, or the obstructive hydrocephalus that necessitated the placement of a shunt.

"I've already got a thing in my head," Sarah had complained when they told her about it.

Fred brought a shunt up to her room to show her what it looked like.

"See, it's only a piece of rubber," he said, sliding her fingers over it. "It's a little like cooked spaghetti."

Sarah quieted down, and the procedure took place, giving her some relief until the steady deterioration that had begun a few months ago. She started to experience constant pain, followed by a sharp loss in motor coordination. For a while, Sarah hung on to a meager ability to walk and talk, then she lost even that. A short time later, she could barely swallow or keep her eyes open.

Whenever Sarah looked in the mirror her parents kept by her bed, she saw a face that must have frightened her. Yet she never asked why she looked that way or what was happening. Perhaps she no longer expected to be beautiful; perhaps she no longer expected to live.

Whenever Sarah's moans and cries became too much, Daniel retreated into his den and wept. He had resolved never to let his daughter see him cry.

The Glazers' small house became crowded with home-care equipment—an IV pole and cartons of prefilled IV bags, suctioning equipment, a catheter drainage system, a feeding tube, syringes, dressings, and a wheelchair. The odor of medications even crept in under the door of his den.

Home health nurses showed Daniel and Lila how to change the IV bags, how to empty the urine bag, and how to suction Sarah when fluid accumulated in her throat. But when one nurse suggested that they rent a hospital bed, Lila screamed.

"I won't have it, I won't have such a thing in my house."

Eventually, she acquiesced as it became more and more difficult to get Sarah into a sitting position.

The bed was too big to go through the doorway of her room, so Sarah was moved into the living room along with the rest of the equipment. Drugs, IV bags, and bed liners were piled high in the French Provincial armoire, which Lila, in another life it seemed, had protected with such care. The hospital, where the Glazers had lived intermittently for so long, had come home to them.

The school had come home, too. Lila continued to read to Sarah and to explain math problems when the child seemed interested.

Once there was a crisis when the laptop computer malfunctioned, and Sarah could no longer communicate. She was in a panic, but Naomi thought of the solution.

"We can still talk a little, Sarah," she said. "I'll ask you a question, and if the answer is yes, blink your eyes once, and if it's no, blink them twice."

They went on to elaborate the code, he remembered, with Sarah enjoying the game.

Putting Sarah's bed in the living room proved to have advantages that Daniel hadn't anticipated. Sarah could see out the picture window, and it seemed to keep her connected to life.

Just a few weeks ago, as Halloween approached, she had noticed the carved pumpkin on the steps of the house across the street.

"I want Halloween," she typed on the repaired computer.

Lila went to a party store and bought a Bozo the Clown costume, face paints, and a few cans of Silly String.

Sarah looked on with delight as Naomi and Lila sprayed the living room with the Silly String, transforming the IV pole, the wheelchair, and even the bed itself into gooney-looking monsters. Somehow they got Sarah into the costume, and Naomi painted her sister's face white and added bright red circles and a large, smiling mouth.

By the time Daniel came home, they were all exhausted.

Lila and Naomi were lying on the sofa, buried beneath cob-webs of Silly String. Sarah was alseep, the arm with the IV hanging limply near the edge of the bed, a polka-dot clown hat balanced precariously on her swollen head.

A few weeks later, Sarah was in the hospital, and Fred was trying to tell Daniel that there could be no more Halloweens.

All at once, Daniel saw the Halloween party as a sad cha-rade. What pleasure, after all, could Sarah really have gotten out of it?

An awful phrase elbowed its way into his mind—"quality of life." An impartial observer would have noted that Sarah had precious little of it, but how in the name of heaven could a parent be expected to use *that* to measure whether to want a child to go on living? Easy enough to talk about quality of life when it was someone else's child. For no matter how little was left of Sarah, he wanted her.

Daniel groaned, and the words of the Twenty-third Psalm came to his lips automatically.

"The Lord is my shepherd; I shall not want. Yea, though I walk through the valley of the shadow of death, I fear no harm for You are with me."

Daniel had recited these sentences many times, but now they offered no comfort. He was suspended, as was Sarah, between life and death, deep, deep in the valley of the shadow.

He looked at a shelf of eclectic theological books—Martin Buber, Kahlil Gibran, and a Zen master—through which he had often pored, looking for some word, some direction. Please, he had thought as he turned the pages, let there be something, anything. Now something was coming into con-sciousness, even as he resisted it.

He had a vision of himself cradling a little girl with cork-screw curls, a little girl who could help to bake cakes and sing and ride a bicycle. But as he held her in his arms, the little girl's hair grew limp and her face white. Her body stiffened, and Daniel realized that he was holding a corpse.

Daniel trembled, and he could hear Fred's words: "You have to help her to die."

He opened the door of the den and walked into the living room, taking care not to bump into the medical equipment. Strange how, even with the inconvenience, he had accepted it as a permanent part of his life.

Now he saw that one day soon a van would pull up to the door and men would remove the stuff, item by item, leaving the bed for last. Finally, they would get around to the bed, and struggle to get it through the front doorway and down the steps.

Daniel would have to stand there, his arm around Lila, and watch them do it. And when they were gone, the living room would be very empty, and there would be no Sarah.

He had let himself recognize the words—there would be no Sarah.

Daniel flung himself down on the hospital bed and clutched each side of the mattress, as if he wanted to hold on to it forever. Then, sighing deeply, he relaxed his grip.

CHAPTER 12

"Boy, I sure respect that other surgeon now," Mike Wilson said.

"You should have respected him before. It wasn't an easy tumor to find," Fred replied.

Fred and Mike were sitting in Fred's office, comparing notes after the morning's operation on Leslie Frazier. Mike had been critical of the doctor who had done the initial surgery, arguing that he should have "taken more," but when they opened, they found that the tumor was deeper than the MRI suggested.

Mike looked nonplussed, feeling that he had broken an unspoken rule: "Don't open your mouth until you've been in there."

"Forget about it. You'll learn," Fred said softly.

Mike was a good resident, Fred thought, who was nearing the end of a long, hard road. He'd been through four years of medical school, one year of internship, and now, an intense six-year program in neurosurgery at NYU.

Each year there were about sixty applicants for two positions. It took three full Saturdays to screen the applications, and narrow the number to be interviewed down to thirty.

What was the department looking for? Intelligence, research, top references, of course. But in Fred's view, intangibles counted the most: self-discipline, a certain creative spark—the need to become expert at something—and endurance in the face of fatigue. Just like a quarterback, a resident had to be able to go on through unexpected periods of overtime. "They should all be athletes," Joe Ransohoff had said once. He also listed among his requirements, "the ability to see in three dimensions."

Fred had another important criterion: the capacity to admit an error. "The worst thing you can do is to try to hide a mistake," he told residents routinely. "Hey, everyone screws up once in a while. Face up to it, and go on from there. We learn from our mistakes."

Surgical technique was important, but a lot of it, even the high-tech stuff, could be classified as mere mechanics. It was the head behind the hand that made the difference.

Mike got up and joined a group of residents, fellows, and interns, who were looking at tapes of operations in the rear of the office. One of the fellows came from Turkey, whose government was paying for his course of study. When the man returned home, he would be the first pediatric neurosurgeon in the country.

Jeff Wisoff was explaining some of the aspects of the procedures shown on the tapes. Fred could see his oval-shaped head moving up and down excitedly as he answered questions. Jeff was a thin-faced young man with glasses and a neatly trimmed mustache; he was the father of two young girls. Jeff was as concerned about the human dimensions of his work as he was about the scientific side of it. Jeff had even chosen the medical school he attended, George Washington University in Washington, D.C., because it was humanistically oriented. Fred made no secret of the fact that he considered Jeff one of the smartest people he knew.

The buzz of conversation was steady, but it didn't bother Fred, who welcomed background distractions. He was used to having an entourage nearby, whether in the office, on his rounds, or in the OR.

He got up, restless, and wandered into the outer office.

Rochelle Sedita was on the telephone arguing with the representative of a health insurance company, which had turned down a patient's claim for part of a procedure.

"We sent Dr. Epstein's explanation to you," she said. "On the twenty-fourth of last month. Why don't you see if you can find it?"

As she spoke, tapping a pencil nervously on the table, a small child with a brace on his leg limped into the room. He was one of the children who were receiving rehabilitation therapy on the unit outside.

The boy held out his hand, and Rochelle dropped in a candy from the supply she kept in her desk for these children.

Fred stroked the youngster on the head, then reached into the drawer and took a sweet for himself.

"Anything else to eat?" he queried JoAnn.

"How do you feel about homemade brownies?" she replied.

"I feel great about them. Do you have any?"

JoAnn shoved a box toward him, a gift that had come in the mail from a patient's mother.

"Do you want to dictate an answer to Mr. Thomas and some of these other letter writers?" JoAnn asked.

Mr. Thomas had written after reading about Fred in a magazine. "My daughter, Holly, twenty-three, was operated on for what we thought would be a routine procedure. It turned out to be a living nightmare. The surgeon said she has a terminal tumor, astrocytoma, grade IV, of which 50 to 60 percent was removed. Recently, a fellow at work showed me an article about you. I'm an eternal optimist, and I believe that somehow, somewhere, there must be a new course of action. I hope and pray you'll have a chance to look at the enclosed medical records."

Fred had looked at every nuance on the MRI, but the phrase "grade IV" told the story. The malignancy was advanced and diffuse, spread throughout the brainstem. Nothing could be done for Holly.

The publicity he got was a two-edged sword, Fred reflected. It directed parents to him who wouldn't have known where to get help otherwise, but sometimes it conveyed the impression that he could "work a miracle" on any type of tumor. Unfortunately, that wasn't true. Some tumors, particularly highly malignant ones, were inoperable.

Soon, Fred believed, there would be "new courses of action" to be used on patients like Holly Thomas. They would stem not from advances in surgery, but from new chemotherapeutic drugs and methods of delivery.

In the meantime, Fred had to make himself do the thing he hated most, give bad news to a despairing parent. He struggled through it, avoiding the word "hopeless," which was a word he never used, no matter what the circumstances.

The reply to the next letter brought Fred particular satisfaction. The addressee was Mohammed Khalil Makkati in Beirut, Lebanon. Fred wrote: "Your son has a tumor in an area I call the cervicomedullary junction [the meeting of the brainstem and the spinal cord]. We commonly operate in this area and have had reasonably good results as most of these tumors are not cancerous. I would be more than pleased to accept your son under my care. I will carry out the operation without charging you any fee, and I also can arrange that no other physician charge a fee, if money is a problem for you."

"Is that it?" Fred asked JoAnn.

"Of course not," she answered, shoving a pile of papers and MRIs into his arms. "By the way, the Breakman girl has a cold and her mother's concerned about your doing the surgery now."

"If the mother's nervous, we won't operate, even if the pediatrician's cleared her. Reschedule."

A few minutes later, Fred was on the phone. "Frank, I looked at the MRI. No evidence of a tumor at all." He gazed down at the desk, frowning, chewing slightly at his lower lip. "Sure, sure, we'll talk later. Keep me in touch."

A buzz, and then JoAnn's voice on the intercom: "Can I send in the Buenos Aires people?"

"Sure."

The patient, Christina Fierro, was a chubby toddler with liquid brown eyes. As she sat in her father's lap, Fred moved her legs gently. Turning her over, he ran his hands along the fifteen-inch scar that ran the length of her spine, a testament to previous surgery.

When Mr. Fierro released her, Christina crawled crab-style across the room, babbling, delighted to be free. She suffered from spina bifida, a congenital birth defect in which two or three of the vertebrae in the back fail to develop, leaving a section of the spinal cord exposed. Depending on the severity of the disorder, a child's legs may become completely or partially paralyzed. There are often bowel and bladder problems, too, and mental handicaps.

The incidence of spina bifida is about one case per thousand babies born. Surgery to close the opening is most effective in the first few days of life, before the spinal cord becomes damaged further.

Christina had already undergone one operation, and Mr. Fierro wondered if another was advisable.

"No," Fred said, shaking his head. Christina had good coordination in one leg, and it was likely that with physical therapy, she would learn to walk with the assistance of a walker. Her mental development seemed to be normal.

Further surgery at this point would do little good, Fred explained, and could even cause greater damage. He thought it a bad idea to manipulate a spinal cord that was already fragile from being "tethered," a condition in which the tip of the spinal cord gets stuck to the membranes that surround it.

"Christina's doing remarkably well," he concluded. "If she starts to regress, loses coordination, for example, then we'll think about doing something. But that may never happen."

Mr. Fierro looked disappointed. The surgeon in Buenos Aires had given him the same advice, but he had hoped that Fred, with his reputation as a "miracle worker," would be able to come up with another answer.

A man of extreme wealth, Mr. Fierro was accustomed to getting what he wanted, but his daughter's illness had changed all that. For the first time in his life, he couldn't control a situation to his liking, and it was tearing him apart.

He walked over to the window and stared out at the heliport, while Mrs. Fierro dressed Christina.

"He wants to have a perfect child, Doctor," she said. "He doesn't see that she is already perfect."

She spoke with such love and simplicity that Fred felt a lump in his throat.

After the Fierros left, Fred wondered why Mr. Fierro couldn't see the vibrancy in his daughter's eyes. She was basically a healthy little girl, with a full life ahead of her. Many parents who came into his office would have been grateful for such a prognosis. For Mr. Thomas, it would have been an answer to his prayers. The grass was always greener, the saying went, but on Fred Epstein's side of the fence, no grass was truly green, just varying shades of gray. Those parents who could learn to accept the gray were the fortunate ones.

Fred turned to the pile of letters on his desk. One was from a regional magazine.

"Dear Dr. Epstein," it read. "Enclosed is a prepublication copy of an article on the Guardians of Hydrocephalus, in which there are several references to you. Please look it over, and if you have any comments, let us have them within a week."

The article had to do with a support group for the parents of hydrocephalic children that Fred had been instrumental in forming.

Hydrocephalus, the abnormal accumulation of cerebrospinal fluid, or CSF, within the ventricles of the brain, is one of the most common "birth defects," affecting over ten thousand babies each year. Many years ago, it was taken for granted that such children would have a shortened life span, characterized by mental and physical retardation, but now, thanks to new diagnostic scans and the insertion of shunts, the long-term survival rate is 85 percent.

However, miraculous as they have proved to be, shunts *can* develop problems.

"Why can't you just put a needle in the baby's head and take the damn fluid out?" a mother once asked Fred after a shunt incident.

He patiently explained that draining the CSF would not, unfortunately, keep the liquid from continuing to accumulate. With hydrocephalus, there was no cure, just living with the shunt. The problem was that constant watchfulness tended to make parents overprotective.

Fred remembered one mother who wouldn't allow her nine-year-old to go to the playground.

"The shunt's made of siliconized rubber, not glass," Fred told the woman kindly. He went on to explain that there was a slight risk of injury in activity. "But isn't it worth it to go for a normal life?"

She looked at him quizzically, but tried his approach, allowing her son to attempt to do first one thing and then another, until she realized he would survive. A few years later, she told Fred that the boy was playing baseball, wearing a helmet, and even though his left hand shook a little, getting his share of hits.

"These parents need help in letting the kids leave the nest," Jeff Wisoff, who handled a great deal of the shunt work in the practice, once explained to a group of residents.

Moral support was part of the answer, not only from physicians, but from other parents. In the late 1970s, a group of parents in the New York metropolitan area started the Guardians of Hydrocephalus with Fred's help. "You have to let the world know what your problems are," he insisted.

Since that time, the ideas this group set into motion have been adopted by other families. Many times Fred and Jeff Wisoff have flown thousands of miles to talk with interested groups, speak at their seminars, approve educational materials, and attend their fund-raisers.

The article Fred had been asked to review primarily concerned an interview with a member whose son Philip had been a patient since infancy.

"One time when Phil was four," the woman recalled, "he wanted to bring his monster truck with him to the operating room. The nurse said no, and he raised an awful fuss. Fred said he could bring it on the gurney with him. They put Philip to sleep on the gurney, and the truck never got into the operating room, of course, but Fred knew it would comfort him to have it."

Fred smiled. He could remember prying the tiny fingers loose from the enormous Tonka toy, which took up just as much room on the gurney as the boy did.

He read further. "Fred's always been there for me. I phoned him once after he had left the office for Fire Island. He called me back collect from the expressway. He apologized for calling collect, but he had no change. He said he was turning the car around and would meet me at the hospital."

It had been an emergency; Philip had developed a sudden blinding headache that signaled the need for an immediate shunt replacement. Philip had been operated on so often that the mere thought of the hospital made him hysterical. By the time Fred got there, three nurses were trying to hold him down to give him a shot. Fred managed to calm him down a bit.

"I don't want the operation, Dr. Epstein," he sobbed.

"Hey, pal. You know it will make your head stop hurting," Fred comforted him.

"When my head is wrapped up, the other kids make fun of me," Philip said.

"They're dopes," Fred stated emphatically.

Philip laughed, and started to relax.

Just a few weeks ago, Fred had seen Philip at one of the Guardians' dinner dances, events that Fred never missed. Phil was now twenty-five years old, running his own business, and living a life that his mother described as "ninety percent normal."

Also at the dinner dance was Martha Simpson, a thirty-six-year-old woman whom Fred called his "geriatric patient." Martha's hydrocephalus wasn't discovered until she began to have severe headaches in her early twenties. That's when Fred put in a shunt.

A few years later, Martha said that she and her husband wanted to start a family.

"Is it possible?" she asked.

Jeff Wisoff didn't see why she and her husband shouldn't try. A short while later, Martha became one of the first female hydrocephalics to become pregnant.

Throughout the pregnancy, Jeff monitored her for increased intracranial pressure, which did, indeed, occur. Martha's symptoms were treated by bedrest, fluid restriction, and the use of diuretics. She was able to deliver the baby vaginally, with the aid of a forceps, so that the second stage of labor—the pushing part—was shortened, thus keeping the increase in cerebrospinal fluid pressure minimal. Throughout the pregnancy, no major problems developed with Martha's shunt.

The last time Fred had examined Martha, her four-year-old daughter was curious about the shunt, so he gave her one of her own to take home.

How strange, he thought. The device that saved the mother's life had become a toy for her child. How triumphant, too, that a woman who would not have survived in earlier decades had lived to become a mother.

Fred wrote, "Good piece, no comments," on the top of the article and put it in the return envelope.

Rochelle poked her head in the door. "The Boss is here," she said with a smile, but before Fred had a chance to respond, "the Boss," Miriam Lubling, was already in the room.

Wearing a white blouse and black suit that matched her coal-black hair, she looked like the sedate Orthodox Jewish woman she was, but her appearance belied the fact that the sixtyish Mrs. Lubling was actually a human dynamo and self-appointed angel of mercy. Twelve years ago she had founded Bikur Cholim, an organization dedicated to saving sick children, no matter where in the world they lived.

If she "heard about" a poor child with a brain tumor in Brazil or England or Israel, the organization would pay to fly the child to Fred.

"Every doctor I bring children to is the biggest and the best," she would declare with pride.

The hospital had given Mrs. Lubling an identification pin as well as carte blanche to wander around to check on "her" children. Fred never knew when she would appear, but he was always delighted to see her. She brimmed with life.

"I got a call from Venezuela," she announced.

Fred said nothing. With Mrs. Lubling, there was no need to ask questions; the answers would come of their own accord.

"The parents have no money, and the doctor says it's a bad one." She was referring to a tumor. "He's sending the records. I said I would pay. When do you think you can fit it in, the operation?"

She had fiddled with his OR schedule more than once. "It's not easy to be a nudge," she told Rochelle on one occasion, "but look, it gets things done."

"I want to see the records first," Fred replied.

"But you'll do it soon?"

"Yes, boss," Fred said.

Mrs. Lubling said that she would check the airline schedules.

"By the way, how's my little boy from Ecuador?"

Mrs. Lubling had paid the airfare for Carmen and Luis to come to New York, and she counted him among "her" children.

She listened thoughtfully as Fred explained the situation.

"Something makes the mother worried," Mrs. Lubling concluded solemnly, "not only the tumor."

Her intuition matched his own.

Later that afternoon, as he made rounds at dusk, he thought

about what Mrs. Lubling had said. He found Carmen Olmedo asleep in a chair in Luis's room. He stood over her, not daring to wake her, but wishing there was some way of breaking through to her.

"She needs her rest," a voice said behind him.

Lila Glazer looked as if she needed rest, too. There were deep circles under her eyes, yet there was something different about her today, an air of peace.

"Thank you for talking with Daniel," she said. "I think he understands now."

"And you?" Fred asked.

"I understand, too."

Fred held her tight in his arms, neither of them speaking for a few seconds. Then he turned and walked quickly out of the room.

CHAPTER 13

F red couldn't get Luis Olmedo off his mind. Time was ticking away, and he was no closer to understanding Carmen Olmedo than he had been a few days before. Her attitude seemed to fly in the face of what was normal for a parent. Most parents wanted to play out every bit of hope, grateful that a spinal cord astrocytoma could now be operated on at all.

Fred thought back a decade or so to the time when he first imagined the possibility of such an operation.

It had begun with a dental appointment.

Fred was sitting in the dental chair, where it seemed to him he spent too much time altogether, the result of a poor gene pool as far as teeth were concerned.

The dentist was hovering over him with the dental Cavitron, when Fred, who had witnessed Joe Ransohoff's work with the Cavitron on brain tumors, envisioned the instrument being used on the spinal cord. He could see it working its way through the narrow tissue, vaporizing a tumor bit by bit and suctioning it off, just as the tartar on his teeth was now being eliminated.

It was an odd juxtaposition, the kind that his father had always encouraged him to pursue. "You've got to let your mind float free," Joseph Epstein said, "and the ideas will come." It didn't matter how ridiculous an idea might seem at first, it had to be explored. "You must be willing to look like an ass, if you're ever going to look like a genius," was an Epstein dictum; so Fred was always ready to embrace a "eureka" idea, even if it proved to be a dud later on.

But now he knew for certain that he had the genuine article—a truly important insight. He bolted out of the chair, knocking a tray of instruments to the floor. Apologizing to the dentist, he hurried out, reaching the street just as a taxicab pulled up to the curb.

Fred stood by impatiently as the passenger, an elderly woman, fumbled to get her packages together.

"Allow me to help," he called out, opening the door and offering her his hand. The woman alighted, amazed at such unexpected gallantry.

"It's an unbirthday present," Fred exclaimed, climbing into the taxi himself.

As the cab inched its way through crosstown traffic, Fred went over and over the idea. "It's so simple," he murmured.

"Are you talking to me, buddy?" the driver asked as they arrived at the hospital.

Fred took the elevator to Joe Ransohoff's office on the eleventh floor.

"I know how to get to astrocytoma spinal cord tumors," he announced, explaining that the Cavitron could liquefy and suck out the tumor without destroying the cord.

"You could also do tremendous damage," Ransohoff replied. "Suck out the cord itself."

"Not if we do it right," Fred argued. "And we'd be going for a cure, not just tumor management until the kid died."

Ransohoff leaned back in his chair and placed his stocking feet on the desk.

"Fantastic," he said, after considering for some time. "Do it."

Others in the department urged Fred to try the procedure on laboratory animals first. But there were children waiting, children who had nothing to lose by having the operation. Spinal cord tumors in children are extremely rare, accounting for only 5 to 10 percent of pediatric tumors of the central nervous system; they often meant certain death.

The first patient was Steven Benson, whose parents said, "Go ahead," when Fred explained that he would be doing something entirely new. After the operation, Fred paced nervously until the call came from the recovery room: Steven had moved his legs; later he would recover completely.

Word of Fred's "radical" surgery began to spread, even though he had yet to publish anything about it. Among those who heard about it was another physician at NYU Medical Center, whose four-year-old grandson suffered from such an "inoperable" tumor.

Fred's successful 1981 operation on the boy, nicknamed "Aaron Alligator," after his favorite character in a Dr. Seuss book, was written up a few months later by John Pekkanen in the *Reader's Digest*.

Then the phones began to ring. One of the parents who found Fred as a result of the article was Jane Thurston, an insurance agent in Eastbourne, England. It was her determination in getting in touch with Fred that would ultimately save her little boy's life.

Julian Thurston, seven years old, had been diagnosed with a spinal tumor. An exploratory myelotomy, an opening of the spinal cord, showed that the tumor was an extremely large astrocytoma, extending six inches down his back.

"We're sorry, Mrs Thurston. These types of tumors are

inoperable," one of Julian's doctors on the National Health Service said.

"Isn't there another doctor you can send me to?" she asked, wondering whether the service's notorious bureaucracy was making it difficult to get the needed care.

"Sadly, no," the doctor replied.

The only treatment he could offer was radiation therapy, which he admitted would stunt Julian's growth.

"Then there'll be no radiation," said Jane Thurston emphatically.

A short time later, the Thurstons learned that the radiation treatment would not have saved Julian's life, merely prolonged it.

Jane was in despair. Seven-year-old Julian had been forced by pain to give up his favorite activities, soccer, swimming, singing in the school choir, and playing the violin. Sunken and ashen-faced, he spent most of his time at home, playing with his pet rabbit, Spotty. Clearly, further deterioration and paralysis were not far off.

Then a close friend spotted the *Reader's Digest* article about Aaron Alligator. Within hours, Jane was pestering one of Julian's doctors to contact Fred J. Epstein at New York University Medical Center. The doctor opined that the article was probably "blowing things out of proportion," but she kept after him until he agreed to make the call.

"Send Julian to New York as quickly as possible," Fred advised.

After he learned that Mr. Thurston was a London cab driver, Fred said he would waive his fee. But since the Thurstons would not be covered by health insurance in the United States, the hospital fees would be substantial. For starters, they would have to pay $7,000 when Julian was admitted.

Jane was desolate. The only possibility of saving Julian's life seemed to be slipping out of her grasp. Then Pam Cradduck, an old friend, showed up with the money. She had been saving it to pay off her mortgage.

"Take it," she said to Jane. "I know you would have done the same for me,"

Jane Thurston took her son to New York.

Fred fell in love with both of them immediately. Julian, in spite of his pain, was adorable—big eyes, tentative smile, and a soft, shy voice. Jane, a handsome woman with classic features, spoke in gentle British tones, determined to keep her fear from her son.

To Fred, she looked incredibly brave, a soldier in a simple skirt and blouse with a Peter Pan collar. Julian had Mummy and his yellow teddy bear to keep him company through the ordeal, but Jane was all alone.

She listened carefully as Fred explained the surgery. The tumor, he said, was buried inside the spinal cord, rather like lead inside a pencil. Because the tumor was fixed to the adjacent normal tissue, pulling it out with conventional instruments would also remove that healthy tissue. Instead, Fred would make an incision in the cord and using the Cavitron, go between the nerves to remove the tumor from the inside out, leaving normal tissue undisturbed. He didn't tell her he would have to do everything perfectly; one false step and the damage would be irreparable.

Jane Thurston remained composed, nodding her head to show that she understood him. For all her gentleness, Fred realized that she would do anything to save her son. Nothing would stand in her way—distance, money, the National Health Service. She had made the improbable probable.

Neither Fred nor Jane had any idea of the attention the operation would attract, even though the media had been alerted that a surgical breakthrough would take place at NYU Medical Center the next day. For the first time, Fred would be using the Cavitron in combination with the carbon dioxide laser, which had just come on the market. He would remove the bulk of the tumor with the Cavitron, and use the laser for the "mop-up" work. Ultrasonic dissection had come of age.

On January 20, 1982, Julian Thurston was transported to the sixth floor operating room. After being anesthetized, he was rolled on his stomach, and the upper part of his body placed on two chest rolls. IV lines, arterial monitoring lines, and leads to monitor the evoked potentials were placed on his body. Then his back was shaved, made sterile by the application of Betadine, and draped for the procedure.

Using magnifying loupes to enlarge the view four times, Fred made the skin incision from the ninth thoracic vertebra to the second lumbar vertebra, exposing the dura mater, the tough gray-colored membrane that protects the spinal cord. Using first a knife, then scissors, he cut through the dura to reach the cord itself. Large, self-retaining retractors had been placed along the lines of the incision to hold back the skin and keep the bone exposed. Fred deepened the incision in the spinal cord until he could see the reddish-gray tumor.

He placed an ultrasound probe on the spinal cord to assess the tumor's path and to check for the presence of cysts in the cord itself.

Starting at the rostral end of the tumor, the part closest to Julian's head, Fred aspirated it with the Cavitron, occasionally using the bipolar unit to control small amounts of bleeding.

Each time he evacuated a cyst, a small amount of yellowish fluid would become visible, then get flushed away by the Cavitron.

Next, Fred aspirated the caudal end of the tumor, the part closest to Julian's feet, evacuated a small cyst, and continued working his way upward, destroying the tumor, until only normal tissue was visible. Progress was made by millimeters. By the time Fred stepped back from the operating table, his shoulders aching and his spirits soaring, Julian had been in the OR for eight hours.

A few minutes later, Fred took Jane to the recovery room. They watched as Julian came out of the anesthetic and smiled at his mother. When Fred asked him to wiggle his toes, he complied immediately. A short time later, a pathology report would confirm that the tumor was benign. Fred was thrilled. For him, Julian was a big "save," a child that no one else would or could operate on.

That evening, word of Julian's successful operation was on all the major news shows in the New York City area. Viewers saw a smiling Fred using the pencil analogy to explain how the tumor could be removed, clips of the operation, and Jane Thurston, still impeccably calm. "We contacted Dr. Epstein, and he said that he could do it," she explained simply in one interview.

Fred had, indeed, "done it," and New York City fell in love with the little English boy whose mother had, fortunately, found the one doctor in the world who could save his life.

On television Julian said that he would like to receive some get-well cards from American kids. Thousands of children responded until there was no room on the walls of Julian's room for all of the cards. He got other things, too—an E.T. doll, a Pac-Man set, and a baseball cap from the team of a school in Manhattan, which he wore as much as he could.

Asked what he thought of the operation, Julian replied, "I don't know. I was asleep when it happened."

Happy as the Thurstons were, the surgery didn't end their problems. The hospital costs were piling up, and Jane promised that if she had to she would sell her house to cover them.

As for Julian, he missed his father, Ron, and his thirteen-year-old sister, Claire.

Fred notified the TV stations, determined to have the family's plight publicized. The Metropolitan Taxi Cab Board of Trade, learning that Ron Thurston was a cabbie, raised money for Ron and Claire to come to New York.

"God bless 'em," Ron said as he hugged his little boy close.

Having the family together hastened Julian's recovery; of that, Fred was certain. Ten days after the operation, the boy was discharged, still in a wheelchair. Fred was hopeful, he told Jane, that the tumor was cured. Some fragments had been left behind, but he thought they would remain dormant or perhaps degenerate as similar fragments do in the brains of children.

If the tumor recurred in a few years, Fred would operate again and follow up with radiation treatment, which was far less likely to harm the spinal cord of an older child.

"But I really think you've seen the last of the tumor," Fred said before the Thurstons left for the airport. Then, turning to Julian, "I'm going to miss you pal. Ilana will, too."

Fred's daughter Ilana, close in age to Julian, had been a frequent visitor and an opponent in endless games of Pac-Man.

The airline gave the Thurstons eight seats so that Julian could sleep. As the plane neared Heathrow, the captain called Jane up to the flight deck and warned her to expect a large crowd of photographers. They were indeed there in droves. The Thurstons pushed Julian's wheelchair through the terminal hurriedly, dodging flashbulbs, well-wishers, and the merely curious.

The next day, as reporters hovered around their small house, the Thurstons found out that their Eastbourne neighbors had been busy raising money to pay the hospital bills. One fund-raiser was a spelling bee, suggested by Julian's headmaster, with sponsors pledging a small amount of money for each word the children could spell correctly. Through this and other community efforts, more than $40,000 was raised.

Jane was overwhelmed, and Ron could barely gasp out his thanks at a school assembly a few weeks later.

As Julian recuperated, his case continued to generate publicity. Some British doctors were defensive about the fact that the Thurstons had had to journey to the United States to have the tumor cured. It was regarded as a slur on the National Health Service.

Had the trip really been necessary?

One surgeon sent a letter to Fred stating that he didn't know what all the "fuss" was about.

"I've done a hundred similar operations," he announced on British television. On further questioning, however, it became clear that he had actually operated on a hundred *spines*, not on the spinal cords, using technology that had been designed fifty years earlier. A few of the tumors might have been ependymomas, a type that is clearly demarcated from the adjacent normal cord, and in most cases can be totally extirpated with surgical instruments. In fact, ependymomas, unlike astrocytomas, had long been recognized as treatable.

Fred couldn't help being amused, but he had a strong enough ego to be annoyed, too. The man hadn't even bothered to find out what type of tumor was under discussion. Like most medical pioneers, Fred thought he deserved credit for his accomplishment.

A few months later, Fred met a prominent British professor of neurosurgery at a meeting of the American Association of Neurological Surgeons.

"So you're the one who was involved in all of that nonsense," the surgeon commented. He went on to say that he had been doing the same operation for years, and without having to use any "fancy" instruments.

"Not another one," Fred thought, spoiling for a fight. "I doubt that you have performed such operations, Doctor. You *could* not, without these instruments," he declared quite firmly.

With that, the professor had what Fred described to Joe Ransohoff as "a small temper tantrum" and stalked off, his dignity barely intact.

While the doctors argued, Julian returned to normal. By Easter, he was back in school and had become "quite cricket mad," Jane reported to Fred. He rejoined the swimming club, and he returned to his violin playing. "I can run fast again now," Julian added in a note. He was still getting letters from children in New York, he said, and so everyone in his class had an American pen pal.

Despite his recovery, Julian needed follow-up care. Children with spinal cord tumors are prone to develop scoliosis, a condition in which the spine becomes curved. They can also develop growth problems.

Julian's pediatrician ordered a brace for him, but Julian balked, even when the doctor told him that Fred wanted him to wear it.

Jane looked for another solution, just as she had when told that nothing could be done for Julian's tumor. Journeying four hundred miles, she found a doctor who used electrical stimulation of the muscles to strengthen the spine. Julian never had to wear the brace.

Two years after Julian's surgery, the division of pediatric neurosurgery was founded at NYU Medical Center, one of the first such divisions in the country, with Fred as its head. The publicity surrounding the operation had been "indispensable," Fred confided to Jane, in focusing on the need for the division. He was grateful to her.

The Thurstons, on their part, had reason to continue to be grateful to Fred: The tumor did not return. Julian went on to win a scholarship to a prestigious school, and he became one of the youngest members of the Eastbourne Symphony Orchestra.

Christmas 1990 was a special one for Fred Epstein. Julian Thurston, sixteen years old, returned to America to give a concert in Fred's honor for young patients at the New York University Medical Center. It was his way of saying thank you.

As children in wheelchairs, parents, and nurses looked on, Julian played a serious piece of music, then responded to demands for Christmas carols. Fred stood in a corner watching, a white medical coat covering his blue scrubs.

"Joy to the world, the King is come, let all the Earth rejoice."

As he listened, Fred could feel the gift he had given Julian coming back to him, surrounding him with love.

Each time he operated on a spinal cord tumor, and he had done many such operations since, Fred thought of Julian. Neurosurgeons are bolstered by their successes as much as they are decimated by failures, and Julian had been a major breakthrough.

Everything he had done for Julian, he ached to do for Luis Olmedo, who had a similar tumor, except that Luis's was malignant. With the passing years, much had improved in technology, and Fred thought his technique had improved, too.

"I'm better now than I was then. I know I am."

He remembered Jane Thurston, and how she had fought her way to him, brushing all obstacles aside. He could see her still, standing over Julian, brushing the hair back from his face, tender and very much alone. The look on Carmen Olmedo's face when she talked to Luis in Spanish was so similar, as was her loneliness.

Fred let the images of the two women float freely in his mind, juxtaposing them, Carmen becoming Julian's mother for the moment, and Jane the mother of Luis.

All of a sudden, he understood how he could make his way into the heart of Carmen Olmedo.

CHAPTER 14

Fred Epstein looked around him as the participants gathered for the meeting of the tumor board. Jeff Allen, who would run the meeting, was seated at a rectangular table on the right-hand side of the small room, facing the audience. A pleasant-looking man with glasses, he had been a close colleague of Fred's for fifteen years.

Jeff was one of ten or so pediatric neurooncologists in the country, a leading expert in the difficult specialty of administering chemotherapeutic drugs to children, and a highly caring person. It was Fred who had convinced Jeff to leave his post at Memorial Sloan-Kettering Cancer Center several years ago and join the staff at NYU. He had provided chemotherapy for many of Fred's patients, including Luis Olmedo.

Jeff waited patiently for order to settle on the small, crowded room, whose occupants included pediatricians, neurosurgeons, pathologists, oncologists, and endocrinologists from neighboring institutions as well as from NYU.

These professionals met regularly to present difficult cases of their own and to hear presentations of colleagues' cases.

They could also present cases from physicians in other places—small towns, for example—who needed help with decisions and who had sent along their records, X rays, and scans. The goal was to get input, particularly from representatives of other specialties, on this "high-powered" board.

The meeting was, in effect, a medical think tank and brainstorming session. The discussions were lively, and sometimes competitive—a shouting match and a support session all at once. Medical students and residents, required to attend, stood in the back of the room, eager for both knowledge and fireworks. Fred noticed that Rick Abbott was standing there, too, immaculately attired in a sport jacket and trousers that might have been featured in *Gentlemen's Quarterly* magazine.

Rick was the junior member of the practice, having joined Fred four years previously, after completing a fellowship. Rick had made a choice, he told Fred, between his "beloved mountains" of Colorado, where he came from, and pediatric neurosurgery, which had brought him to New York to work with Fred. Now, though Rick might look like a native New Yorker, Fred knew how much he longed for the quieter, more tranquil environment that suited his nature.

A fellow—a doctor taking a year of advanced training in his field—would present the cases at the tumor board. He had been seated at the table with Jeff Allen. Now the fellow stood up and adjusted the blackboard, which would soon be covered with ideas and options.

"Hi, Fred," said a voice behind him. Fred turned around and recognized an oncologist he had known for a long time. He couldn't for the life of him, though, remember the man's name.

"Hello, my friend," Fred responded, using the pat phrase for cover.

Whenever this kind of lapse occurred, Fred felt a surge of

uneasiness, an anxiety that stemmed from his fear of Alz-heimer's disease, the disorder that had overtaken his mother, changing her from a competent, hard-driving professional into a woman who could not recognize her own sons.

For Fred, it was the most terrible transformation that could be imagined, and he saw signs of it in himself around every corner. No matter that he had *never* been any good at re-membering names, a fact his staff teased him about constantly. Ridiculous, he chided himself. The guy's name will come to me in just a few minutes, or maybe a few hours.

In the meantime, he turned around and murmured a greet-ing, hoping the man wouldn't notice that Fred wasn't using his name.

Fred shifted uneasily in his chair. His nervousness wasn't abating. He regretted having promised Daniel he would bring Sarah's case before the board. When the fellow presented her case, the course of action might seem obvious to the others— provide supportive care and allow the patient to die. There were several people in the room who would be aghast at Fred's discussing the case at all, ready to stick pins in him. Well, let them, Fred thought. It's a good thing I don't mind sounding like a fool. And perhaps there was something to be learned, after all. For deep in his heart, Fred wasn't truly prepared to give Sarah up, something he had been feeling even as he told Daniel Glazer that was what they would probably have to do.

A part of Fred was still wearing blinders where Sarah was concerned, blinders created by years of attachment. Fred had a special attachment to all his patients, but Sarah fell into that extraordinary category of those whom he truly loved. With these patients, it was particularly difficult, even for a doctor who walked with death daily, to face reality.

He remembered Bonita Jeffers, a beautiful sixteen-year-old,

who was a genuine friend as well as a patient. Fred enjoyed talking with her about books and boys and, particularly, about her plans for the future. He was thrilled when she was accepted for early admission to Princeton, but Bonita never got there, because her tumor recurred. For months Fred told himself that the tumor was benign and that she would live, even as the pathology reports advised differently. The thought of going to her funeral was too horrible to be borne.

When Bonita died, Kathy was out of town, and Fred had to take the kids to a family event. He had a limousine waiting for him, but traffic was heavy, and he arrived at the funeral home just as the mourners were filing out. He felt terrible, and he always would.

Sarah's funeral was something he refused to imagine. That was why he had to bring up her case. Perhaps someone else would have an idea. Perhaps there was some experimental treatment he hadn't heard about.

Fred brought himself to attention sharply, realizing that he had missed the beginning of a presentation. The case involved an infant with a malignant brain tumor. The child was too young for radiation therapy—it would affect her skeletal development and her intelligence—and chemotherapy tended to destroy bone marrow. So the oncologist was discussing a fairly new option called "bone marrow rescue."

This course of action involved withdrawing the bone marrow, subjecting the patient to enormous amounts of chemotherapeutic drugs, then putting the bone marrow back into the body. A significant number of kids treated with this technique seemed to respond, though there were no five-year survival rates as yet.

There were substantial drawbacks to the treatment. It made the child sick as hell and, because the immune system became compromised, the patient had to remain in isolation for three weeks. Often, one or both of the parents went into isolation too, scrubbing and donning gowns before being allowed to be with their child. Not a pretty prospect, but the options for this particular case were extremely limited.

An oncologist, a pathologist, and a neurologist discussed the outlook.

"It's God-awful, but it might work," one of them commented.

"We don't have any meaningful survival statistics," another put in.

"Well, then exactly what *would* you do?" the third challenged, a bit testily. The air in the room had become electric.

Fred leaned forward with sheer pleasure. He loved being part of this creative process, loved the debate, the suggestions, even the touches of collegial acrimony. It plugged into his need to explore, to learn about every side of an issue.

Yet few who knew Fred as a student could have imagined him here, today, a major authority in a major medical center. In college his grades could most charitably be described as average, and in chemistry, they were abysmal. "Well, there goes medical school," one of Fred's friends said when the chemistry grades were posted.

But Fred was determined to become a physician. He applied to Albert Einstein Medical School, the University of Chicago, and NYU, and got turned down by all of them.

"You don't belong in this medical school," the dean of NYU Medical School said emphatically at Fred's interview. "The academic record shows that you're emotionally unstable."

Fred didn't think he was unstable, just a different sort of learner. With his father's influence, he got admitted to New York Medical College, then called Flower Fifth Avenue. If he hadn't been accepted, he planned to become a social worker, and in a way, he *had* become a kind of social worker.

You don't really have to be brilliant to be a doctor, Fred thought, just caring, focused, and very knowledgeable about the area in which you work.

Fred had imagined that psychiatry would be his area of knowledge, but by his third year of medical school, he knew it was neurosurgery. Neurosurgery, he discovered while on a one-month rotation in the department, had everything—excitement, risk, glamour; for Fred, it represented the top of the medical pantheon.

From those heights, he could issue a reply to everyone who had downgraded him, including the dean: "See, I made it—and I fit in real well on the top of the mountain."

"We'll be here till the cows come home," a voice said. Fred realized that the discussion about the first presentation was still going on. Finally, the board came to a conclusion, deciding that the pediatric oncologist presenting the case should proceed with the bone marrow rescue.

Next on the agenda was the case of a four-year-old boy who had been operated on by a pediatric neurosurgeon at another hospital for a ganglioglioma of the spinal cord. The pathologists were not completely sure if the tumor was benign or malignant. In some cases, a definite diagnosis is very difficult. Jeff Allen placed the MRI scan in the large viewer at the front of the room so that everyone could see the tumor, which was extremely bulbous and extended from the ninth thoracic vertebra to the conus, the coneshaped lower end of the spinal cord.

Since the tumor was not definitely malignant, the question was whether or not the child should receive radiation therapy. At one time, such treatment would have been administered fairly automatically, but now it was not always recommended. This is because physicians are aware of the serious side effects of the treatment: Radiation could permanently impair the child's growth and damage the spinal cord.

A recent study of thirty tumors similar to the one exhibited by this patient suggested a strong likelihood of recurrence.

"I'd do nothing," one physician suggested.

"Based on what?" another asked.

"The child's age and the fact that the pathologist's report found the neoplasm to be of 'low to moderate cellularity.' A high-celled tumor would be more likely to recur."

"There's not a lot of evidence that radiation treatment is effective with gangliogliomas," Fred offered.

"I wouldn't just watch if it were my patient," said an oncologist. "After all, what are we talking about here—thirty cases?"

Perhaps there were others, a neurosurgeon suggested, and began to review a number of his own cases involving astrocytomas, but none of them concerned the spinal cords of young patients, the latter being the subject of this particular tumor board. The cases were interesting, but rather off the track, Fred thought.

Kids are different, he reflected, with a different sort of biology. When it comes to tumors, one can be more surgically aggressive with children, since they heal better than adults.

In the case under discussion, the surgeon had removed just about all of the tumor, something he wouldn't have been able to do with an adult, because of the greater danger of damage to the cord.

The biggest difference between children and adults, in Fred's mind, was the simple fact that kids weren't meant to have life-threatening diseases. A young life, ripped out almost as soon as its roots had taken hold, was an anomaly he could never accept.

Because kids were different, Fred and other neurosurgeons

who specialized in children—40 out of the 3,500 neuro-surgeons in the country at the time—formed the American Society of Pediatric Neurosurgery in 1978. However, the American Board of Neurosurgery wasn't happy with the society's recommendation that physicians be required to have specialized training in order to be recognized as pediatric neurosurgeons. Certification standards of this sort, the board claimed, would fragment the profession. But Fred and the others felt a strong need to be recognized as a subspecialty.

He remembered the sense of accomplishment he felt when the neurosurgeons gathered for a meeting on the island of St. Maarten in the Caribbean, intent on translating concept into reality, no matter how exalted the opposition.

Everything had to be invented from scratch. For example, what exactly was a pediatric neurosurgeon? They decided it was someone who performed a minimum of two hundred operations on kids each year. Later, there would be other requirements, such as a year's training in pediatric neurosurgery after a neurosurgery residency. As for membership in the new organization, it would be by invitation only. A journal? Of course. One would be started within the year, and a conference was planned, too.

One evening, Fred went out for a sail by himself. The water was totally calm, the sun had dissolved into a blazing ribbon a short time earlier, and now it slipped, strand by strand, into the sea. The sense of satisfaction Fred felt was total. He had seen the birth of something new, and he himself was something new—a pediatric neurosurgeon. He had been drawn to neurosurgery by an instinct and to children by a deep passion. Over time, he discovered how the two, his need and his love, fit together, and he had begun to see what was required for the future.

This day, it had all been put together. He was lucky, terribly lucky, not only in his work, but in his family. "Thank you, God," Fred whispered. When he got back to the hotel, he threw his arms around Kathy, who had accompanied him on the trip. "Let's send a postcard to the kids," he said.

Now he smiled just thinking of it and wondered if anyone at the tumor board was looking at him strangely. No such thing; they were all still absorbed in the debate over the follow-up treatment for the spinal cord ganglioglioma.

The blackboard was covered with writing, a list of options written down by the fellow, based on the group's suggestions.

"What do you say, folks?" came a voice from the rear. "It's time to cut bait."

A few of the participants looked annoyed, but Jeff Allen urged a decision, noting that they still had a full agenda ahead. The board arrived at a consensus: Pursue a course of "watchful waiting," with a follow-up MRI in a few months' time. The decision made Fred a trifle uncomfortable; he feared that the tumor would recur, but it did seem that the best choice had been made under the circumstances.

The next case was a truly tough one. The patient was a sixteen-year-old boy who had grown more than fourteen inches in less than two years, to a height of six feet six inches. At first, his parents were unconcerned, since the father was well over six feet, but during a routine examination, an orthopedist noticed the boy's enlarged hands and feet, a sign of endocrine dysfunction. An endocrinologist diagnosed gigantism—the patient had highly elevated amounts of growth hormone—and ordered an MRI, which revealed a pituitary tumor, a large mass that extended beyond the edge of the skull into the sinus cavity.

The tumor's location suggested that it might not be resectable, but the neurosurgeon whose case it was had been able to perform the operation through the sphenoid bone at the base of the skull.

The fellow passed around a photograph of the patient before the operation. It showed an awkward, gangling young man with a baseball cap on his head, his trousers at least two inches too short, his face distorted by an enlarged nose and jaw. His shoe size was probably thirteen or larger, the fellow commented.

Poor kid, Fred thought.

The boy seemed to be growing out of his skin, and without the surgery he would have reached a height of up to eight feet and would have died, inevitably, of circulatory problems.

Even with the tumor gone, however, the condition of gigantism remained. The overproduction of growth hormone had been reduced, but it hadn't been controlled.

What to do next? The growth plates, the areas between the long bones of the arms and legs where longitudinal growth takes place, had to be closed. Could this be accomplished surgically?

Perhaps. No one in the room was an orthopedist, but a number of people believed it was possible. Another option was the administration of testosterone, the male hormone, known to aid in closing growth plates.

To prevent recurrence of the tumor, an oncologist recommended radiation therapy as well.

"Radiation could create secondary tumors," someone pointed out.

"That was one of my problems with it," commented the neurosurgeon presenting the case.

The oncologist shook his head. "With something like this, you've got to pull out all the stops," he said.

As suggestions came thick and fast, Fred reflected that this was the glory of the tumor board—it provided a truly multidisciplinary approach to problems, without the physician's having to call in other specialists for "consults." It was also a good place to vent doubts, as the neurosurgeon had done when he voiced hesitancy about the radiation therapy.

Fred began to feel a little more comfortable about having Sarah's case aired.

In the meantime, he found the board's decision on the gigantism complete and ingenious: Consult with an orthopedist to determine if the growth plates could be closed surgically—if not, administer testosterone; begin radiation therapy; and start a course of sandostatin, a drug that would lower growth-hormone levels.

The fellow inserted some scans in the viewer for the next case. It concerned "an eleven-year-old white female, who first presented with a highly malignant bifrontal tumor, at six months of age." He went on to review the patient's nine major operations, four hemorrhages into the tumor, chemotherapy and radiation treatments, and the insertion of a shunt. The patient was almost totally paralyzed, aphasic, and experiencing problems in swallowing.

Jeff Allen looked at Fred expectantly, and Fred realized, with some degree of shock, that the case under discussion was Sarah's.

Hearing her spoken about in this cold technological manner was suddenly disturbing. It sounded as if Sarah consisted of only her symptoms. This was the kind of language that got Daniel Glazer and other parents crazed, hearing their children's illnesses translated into medicalese. Yet such words were the lingua franca of the hospital, the way in which medical personnel communicated with one another, perhaps to keep themselves from feeling too much, and Fred had to use them now.

"Despite its malignancy, this tumor acted, at first, like one that was benign," Fred commented. "It was unusual, didn't fit any profile."

"Why wasn't the patient given radiation after you first removed the tumor?" someone asked.

"We had no track record on radiation back then," Fred replied. "It might have destroyed the tumor, but her brain could have been destroyed, too."

Bringing up old history made Fred cringe inside. Had he done everything he could for Sarah, really everything? Then he caught himself. You've got to stop thinking that way, he thought. You know you did your best. Besides, the only thing that counts now is the future.

Someone suggested bone marrow rescue for Sarah.

Then an oncologist began to talk about an experimental regimen in which blood is removed from the body and the white cells are isolated. At this point, the white cells are incubated with interleukin, a biological modifier that turns the white cells into killers that will attack the tumor. After being treated, the cells are infused directly into the tumor beds by means of a shunt.

The regimen, now in its first phase of study, was being tested in the Children's Cancer Study Group (CCSG), a clinical research group in which NYU participated. It was created by the National Cancer Institute, and children who had undergone surgery for their tumors and required chemotherapy were often placed in this group.

These young patients were randomized. Some were given traditional chemotherapy and others given new, untested combinations of drugs that had not previously been used, so that assessments of the new treatments could be compared. What drug a child received was decided randomly, a matter of chance. This was hell to explain to parents. They might be in for a "miracle" or for terrible disappointment and, down the line, the possibility of yet another drug trial that everyone hoped would prove more successful. It was gambling for the highest stakes.

"What about interferon?" an oncologist asked.

He was referring to a protein produced by the body's immune system to fight viral infections. A few years ago, it was thought that interferon might have startling results in reducing tumors, but its value was still unproven.

"How can we use interferon when we're not certain what kind of tumor this is?" Fred asked.

He saw that some members of the board were as committed as he was to coming up with a solution, to extending Sarah's life, if possible. But Fred also saw—with complete clarity—that Sarah was beyond the experimental.

He looked at the rows of X rays and scans displayed in the front of the room. With each operation, the scarring around the original site had become more pronounced, and less penetrable by instruments, blocking the utilization of his own skills. He looked at the thick file on the rectangular table. So many treatments had been tried already. What kind of doctor would want to go on with this?

It was as if the clouds had cleared over a bomb site, revealing the devastation below. Sarah needed peace; she needed rest. Her file had to be closed at last.

Apparently, the other members of the board were coming around to that way of thinking, too. Of the four options listed on the blackboard—conventional chemotherapy, bone marrow rescue, radiation, and nonintervention—the last was receiving the most discussion. Finally, a consensus was reached.

The recommendation was that the poor prognosis be discussed with the parents and that palliative care—keeping

Sarah comfortable through the terminal phase—be initiated. A few board members looked relieved, Fred thought, that they weren't the ones who would have to hold this particular discussion.

Why had he even bothered to bring up Sarah's case? Because I'm here on the top of the mountain, and I want to be able to save those I love. Why doesn't being on top mean that I can do that?

Fred shifted back in his chair, knowing that he had to move beyond emotion. He would dictate the board's decision, as was the practice, in memorandum form and show it to Daniel. Words on paper were significant to the rabbi. They were solid and capable of being comprehended, when so much else was not. Then he would do everything he could to help the Glazers as they watched Sarah die.

Behind him, Fred heard someone clearing his throat. He turned and saw Rick Abbott peering at him seriously. As usual, Rick was preparing to choose his words with care. There was a moment of hesitation before he said, "That was a good decision, I think, about the Glazer case."

Fred knew that in his laid-back WASP manner, Rick had intuited Fred's feelings and was offering him support. He nodded at him gratefully.

As he watched Rick walk away, Fred forced himself to stop thinking about Sarah and to go over the condition of some of the other children he was treating. Kevin Dagner was back in Nine East after two days in intensive care, back in the same room with Luis Olmedo. Leslie Frazier, after successful surgery, was recovering in intensive care. Barbie Marting's new shunt was functioning well, and she would be discharged the next day.

As for Luis Olmedo, Fred had put plans into place, through

Miriam Lubling, that might pleasantly surprise his mother, Carmen. For the rest of the tumor board session, he found himself wondering how those plans were progressing.

When the session was over, he returned to room 518, and addressed JoAnn eagerly.

"Did you get the schedule?" he asked.

"Yup," JoAnn replied. "Ecuatoriana Airlines. Nonstop, leaves Guayaquil at two-fifteen P.M., arrives in New York at nine-fifteen P.M. Fare is $966 for an adult. The Boss thinks she can manage it."

Fred considered a moment.

"What does Tania think?" he queried.

"She thinks you're right on target. Getting her husband up here would be just the kind of support Mrs. Olmedo needs."

Fred valued Tania's opinion, even though she and Fred didn't always agree.

When they didn't, she would say, "You don't respect me because I'm a nurse," and he'd quip, "Nope, it's because you're a girl," and they'd both chuckle.

Once, at a staff meeting that involved several departments, Tania had asked Fred why he didn't want to follow her solution to a particular problem.

"It's because you're a girl," Fred remarked, stone-faced.

There was dead silence. No one in the room knew what to make of this seeming insult, so out of character for Fred, particularly since Tania's face remained as blank as his.

The pair left the meeting looking sedate, but when they got back to the office, they sank down on the sofa, collapsed with laughter.

Fred remembered that now, even as he looked at the paper JoAnn handed him with the airline schedule.

With Carmen Olmedo there would be no quips, and

no ease of communication. He would have to make his proposal through Lourdes Suarez, but unless he misjudged the loneliness and fear in Carmen's eyes, there was no reason for her to turn him down. It was time to go into his office and take a close look at Luis's MRI, in preparation for an operating plan.

CHAPTER 15

*T*he schedule on Fred's desk showed that Luis Olmedo's surgery wouldn't take place in OR 11, the operating room Fred preferred, but in OR 10, right next door. As Fred waited to be called down for his part of the operation, he found the room assignment disturbing, a bad omen. He was so accustomed to OR 11 that he could have traversed its terrain in his sleep. There was something about OR 10, however, that always seemed askew. The lighting was just a trifle too bright, the row of screens above the operating table just a touch more difficult to see. It was probably his imagination creating these feelings, but for this operation, everything had to be right. He longed for the comfort of a room that was "home."

He was carrying a heavy emotional burden. Carmen Olmedo had finally agreed to the procedure, yet Fred felt she still had reservations. Apparently, it was the opinion of her husband, Jorge, who had flown in the day before from Guayaquil, that had tipped the scales in favor of the surgery.

Jorge, Lourdes Suarez reported, was the member of the family who had the most confidence in "scientific medicine," whereas Carmen's mother, Mrs. Delgado, who lived with the Olmedos, opposed it.

When Luis first became ill, Jorge had confided to Lourdes, Mrs. Delgado had insisted on consulting a neighborhood "curer," a woman with a reputation for being expert in the ways of folk medicine. The curer gave Luis several massage treatments for "something hard" in his back, followed by herbal medications.

As Luis continued to deteriorate, Mrs. Delgado urged Carmen to return to their native village and seek a more proficient curer. But Carmen demurred. One day, she wrapped Luis in a shawl and carried him to the cathedral in Guayaquil, where she prayed to the Holy Virgin for guidance.

On the way home, she walked past the World Health Organization clinic for the first time. The clinic was run by Donald Brickelmeyer, who talked to Carmen when she came inside. As a result of that meeting, Carmen was soon on her way to New York with Luis, believing that the Virgin was guiding her.

When Luis returned home—apparently cured—Carmen was willing to believe in science. Each yearly check-up made her feel more secure. But that changed this year when she noticed Luis's slight limp was becoming more pronounced. At first, she pushed it out of her mind, pretended the change wasn't happening, and when her mother commented on it, Carmen told her she was mistaken.

When Fred told Carmen the tumor had returned, her confidence in the treatment was shattered. She began to think her mother had been right after all in warning her that the operation wouldn't work. She would return to Ecuador and find yet another curer.

But Jorge, who was more educated than Carmen, supported the second surgery. Luis's illness, he said, was too difficult a thing for a curer to handle. Only Dr. Epstein's type of "magic" could save Luis.

Now, Fred said to himself, old Dr. Epstein has to deliver. He made the final mental preparations for the surgery, drawing out the full measure of his self-confidence. In the OR, there was no room for self-doubt. There one had to be totally strong, arrogant even, the person everyone else depended on.

As Fred waited, Luis Olmedo lay anesthetized on an operating table in OR 10. Hank Squires, a fifth-year resident, was administering the second application of Betadine solution along the center of Luis's back, from the bottom of his neck to the base of his spine. Two applications were necessary because of the strong danger of infection with this type of surgery.

"I sent the bear back upstairs," a circulating nurse said suddenly to Jeff Wisoff, who was in charge of the first part of the operation.

She was referring to a presurgical incident, which had taken place when Luis first arrived in the OR. He was accompanied on the gurney by a teddy bear, purchased for him by Ina Bea Dagner. This broke a rule, frequently reiterated by Tania, against allowing such furry companions in the OR itself, because of the danger of their getting tossed out with the laundry.

The stuffed animal had been handed over to the nurse who made the comment, and now it appeared she had arranged for its transportation back to Nine East.

"Well done," Jeff commented.

Hank and Jeff placed sterile towels around the area in which the incision would be made. Then Hank placed a clear, plastic sheet, the underside covered with sticky material, on Luis's bare skin. The incision would be made first through the clear plastic, rather than the skin itself, another "trick" to hold infection at bay.

"Knife."

A scrub nurse took the instrument from the overhead table and handed it to Jeff, who deftly made an incision from the first thoracic vertebra to the tenth, almost all the way down the spinal column, following the scar of the previous operation. The incision was a shallow one, penetrating just through the skin down to the deep fascia, the bands of connective tissue beneath the skin.

The gateway to Luis Olmedo's spinal cord was open, the first step toward reaching the invader that had insinuated itself within. But this outer bastion, having been taken, needed to be secured.

Jeff placed two self-retaining retractors into the fascia to keep the wound open. Then, using the electrocautery unit, he coagulated the blood vessels.

The operation could proceed only when all bleeding had stopped. A spinal cord operation had to be particularly "dry." Otherwise, visibility would be obscured.

At this point, Fred Epstein arrived quietly in the OR. He stood on a stool behind Jeff, so he could look over his shoulder.

It seemed to be taking an eternity for Jeff to complete the cauterization, Fred thought, for he was eager to engage this particular tumor. He wanted to get all of it out, to eradicate it.

Jeff continued to work in his quiet, methodical way, without the slightest notion of the storm raging inside his partner. Or was he so unaware? Though Jeff was a much more reticent person than Fred, in some ways their personalities were similar enough for Jeff to fit easily inside Fred's skin. He, too, tended to get very involved with families and to agonize over every lost patient. And, like Fred, he was a physician's son who had wanted to be a doctor since childhood.

"I can remember, when I was about four or so, being held

in my mother's arms and looking through my father's copy of *Gray's Anatomy*," Jeff had once told Fred happily.

Fred could visualize the very serious preschooler, eschewing Mother Goose in favor of organs, bones, and muscles.

Well, it had certainly paid off. Jeff, like Rick Abbott, was an excellent surgeon. I've certainly been fortunate in getting both of them to work with me, Fred thought, just as Jeff succeeded in controlling the bleeding.

Next, Jeff had to open the fascia and separate the muscles from the bone that surrounds the spinal cord. He accomplished this by using the Bovie electrocautery knife, which actually stripped the muscle from the bone.

When Jeff finished, the vertebrae of Luis's spine were totally exposed—like those of a fish about to be deboned.

"How are we doing?" Fred asked the anesthesiologist.

"Smooth as silk," the man replied.

Luis's upper body was elevated somewhat, resting on large bolsters, to permit his chest to expand as he breathed. That breathing was done for him by a ventilator, since his own respiratory system had been paralyzed by the anesthetic.

The anesthesiologist continuously checked Luis's respiratory and cardiac functions by means of leads attached to his body. An operation such as this, which would last at least six hours, could put a great strain on the vital systems of a young child, particularly one like Luis who had not been especially well nourished.

"Annie, the Midas Rex, please," Jeff said.

The instrument the scrub nurse handed him was a compact pneumatic drill, which looked rather like a fat pencil. At high speed—sixty thousand revolutions per minute—it had the capacity to cut through bone like butter.

Now, remarkably, the drill would enable Jeff to remove in

one piece the part of the vertebrae called the laminae, which had actually been removed and replaced in the procedure performed on Luis three years ago. He accomplished the maneuver in two stages. First, he made two incisions—one on each side of the bone, dividing it in two. Then, he separated the ligaments beneath the bone from the dura, the membrane that covers and protects the cord itself.

The bone became totally loosened. With Hank's assistance, Jeff lifted it out, all twelve inches of it, and handed the bone to a nurse, who placed it in a pan filled with an anti-infectant. There it would rest until it was put back into Luis's body at the end of the surgery.

Fred, who had been out of the room scrubbing up, returned and stared down at the dura, which bore the scar of the previous surgery. It had also become tissue-thin and compressed, due to the abnormal blood vessels pressing against it. The blood vessels belonged to the malignant tumor.

This dura was going to be exceedingly difficult to open, Fred thought.

Fred proceeded confidently, sustained by the normality of operating room routine. The nurses were the same familiar ones he usually worked with, smart, dedicated, knowledgeable about the most minute part of every piece of equipment in the room, and able to anticipate his every move. There was no question that everything he needed would be handed to him in a second, in the right position, ready to use. Jeff— well, Jeff was like a part of himself, a former resident he had trained and ultimately convinced to join his practice.

Fred placed an ultrasound transducer on the dura, and with that, ultrasound pictures of the tumor appeared on the screens above.

These pictures provided a two-dimensional view, both lateral and cross-sectional, and Fred could see that the tumor was of enormous proportions. Remarkable, he thought, that Luis had shown so few symptoms.

"We didn't get him in here a minute too soon," Fred said through his mask.

Jeff nodded. He was checking the pictures himself, comparing them with the MRI films posted on the walls, and reviewing the details of the operating plan. It was clear to Fred that without this operation, Luis would probably have been dead within months.

A cloud lifted from Fred's mind. He'd been right in stressing the importance of the surgery to Carmen. Every single minute of a child's life counted, he reminded himself. And here, now, he would be extending those minutes, keeping the mechanism of the clock going when it had been so close to running down. No way he'd let that happen, Fred swore, no way.

Lourdes Suarez had once told him a Hispanic legend. Somewhere, there's a cave filled with candles, a candle for the life of each person on earth. Some of the candles are tall, others short and stubby and covered with accumulated tallow. These short candles belong to those without much life left, most of them elderly people. But sometimes, sadly, the short candles are those of children. It's the way fate works things out, Lourdes reported.

Fred found it hard to accept that notion, even though he saw very sick children every day. If only he could find that cave, he would replace each short candle representing a child's life with a tall one. He'd set things right.

He began to talk, with the object of involving Hank and also the medical students, who were crowded around the video monitor. A spinal cord tumor took even longer to remove than a brainstem tumor, and the procedure could be more tedious. Yet constant attention was required because such surgery had to be absolutely perfect—there was no other possibility.

"This is a kid from a slum in Guayaquil in Ecuador," Fred said with urgency. "The place is filled with poverty and disease. He hasn't had many breaks, so let's hope that we can give him a break."

He went on talking, longer than he usually did in these situations. Was he making sense? He didn't care. "There are four older siblings, and an old grandmother, and there's not too much room in the hovel they're forced to live in. But it's a home, and it will be terribly empty if Luis isn't there." And Carmen Olmedo's heart will be broken if something goes wrong.

What was that snatch of prayer attributed to Moses Maimonides, the great Jewish theologian and physician of the twelfth century? "Grant me strength of spirit to faithfully execute my work."

"Strength of spirit" was what he prayed for.

Fred used the ultrasound to identify the top and bottom portions of the tumor. This was important, as he had to make certain these markers could be visualized before attempting to remove the tumor.

"Number eleven," he said.

The blade was in his hand instantly.

He made an incision in the lower end of the dura, and then used a microscissors—a tiny version of a scissors, suitable for such close work—to open it up. It was difficult, since the tumor was pressing against the dura very tightly, rather like a sausage in a casing. Fred moved the scissors along gingerly, his hand so steady it seemed not to be human, but rather an instrument itself.

Jeff retracted—pulled back—the dura with small sutures, which were hung on clamps.

Now part of the reddish-gray tumor became visible. Fred was struck by its abnormality and the insidious degree of spread. There were parts of the tumor on the cord's surface, inside it as well, and extending out from beneath. These were killer cells, and every last bit of them had to be removed to give Luis the best chance possible.

To attack the tumor, Fred first had to perform a myelotomy, an incision down the exact midline of the spinal cord. Generally, the midline had to be painstakingly determined by measuring from the nerves coming out of either side of the cord, but in Luis's case, a three-year-old scar mapped the way.

"Scope on," Fred said. A scrub nurse activated the instrument by turning on a switch.

"Laser, eight watts."

As Fred moved the laser along, Jeff followed close behind, coagulating blood vessels with the electrocautery unit. Their blue gowns touching, each doctor had the same serious expression behind his surgical mask, and they seemed to be moving in tandem—four hands, one mission.

Jeff used a plated bayonet forceps, a flat, knifelike instrument, to separate the edges of the myelotomy, and then he placed traction sutures on clamps along the length of it. There were now at least twenty-five pieces of metal, clamps of various sizes, in the opening in Luis Olmedo's back.

Fred took some biopsies and handed them to a nurse to prepare for the lab. The tumor seemed to be a "bad actor," as the medical phraseology went.

"We'd better get ready for a lot of bleeding," Fred remarked to Jeff and Hank, commenting on the tumor's high degree of vascularity.

Fred zoomed in to ten power with the scope, close to full strength, and began to debulk the tumor, using the Cavitron.

He started to work at the caudal end, the part closest to

Luis's feet, simply because the tumor was most visible here. It was like beginning a long climb up a mountain, the top of which was buried in the clouds. Fred didn't have a complete idea of what lay ahead except that the way would be hard and slow and that the summit had to be reached somehow.

He used the Cavitron in bursts of five to fifteen seconds. Before this operation was over, there would be countless such bursts, each directed with the same care and precision. At no point, until he said "Let's close," could Fred let down his guard.

As he worked, the ultrasound was used intermittently to confirm that the tumor was being removed and to identify the areas where more of it was hidden. With that knowledge, Fred pursued the intruder, and after each "evacuation," a tiny area would fill with blood, as the tumor left its calling card.

That blood had to be stopped. Jeff was at Fred's elbow, cauterizing, irrigating, and filling the area with cottonoid sponges.

It was difficult to keep up with the bleeding, and the blood often obscured Fred's vision, making it difficult to distinguish between tumor and normal tissue. As Fred inched his way up the spinal cord, he hoped the tumor might become less vascular, but it didn't.

Two hours later, he reached the midcord point.

"How much blood have we lost?" Fred asked the scrub nurse, who was measuring the loss by weighing the used sponges.

"About a hundred ccs," she estimated.

Not too dangerous yet, Fred thought. Would it become necessary to transfuse Luis?

"Blood pressure's okay," the anesthesiologist said. "105 over 60."

The tumor looked slightly less vascular ahead, or was that

wishful thinking? Fred considered lowering the power on the Cavitron, in the hope of precipitating less bleeding, but that would also make the instrument less effective. He couldn't afford to leave any tumor behind. There was nothing to do but move ahead.

It seemed to Fred that Jeff looked concerned, his eyebrows furrowed above his mask. Perhaps he would have stopped at this point, but it wasn't his decision, it was Fred's. Anything that went wrong would fall squarely on Fred's shoulders.

Maybe because Fred wanted it so much, the bleeding came under better control as he approached the rostral end of the tumor, the part closest to Luis's head. The top of the mountain had come into view, and Fred felt a sense of relief; but it was short-lived.

"Hold what you're doing, Fred, I'm getting an irregular heartbeat," the anesthesiologist called out. An alarm bell sounded.

Hastily, Fred and Jeff withdrew their instruments from the operating field.

Within seconds, blood pressure had fallen. The anesthesiologist struggled to raise it by pumping a drug into an IV, but to no avail.

Luis was experiencing ventricular fibrillation, independent, random contractions of each ventricular muscle cell. As a result, the ventricles of the heart merely quivered, instead of producing the synchronized contractions necessary to pump blood through the body.

The anesthesiologist got on the intercom. "Cardiac arrest, ten," he said.

"Let's pack up this wound," Fred ordered. Luis would have to be turned on his back so that his heart could be shocked back to life.

Working swiftly, Fred, Jeff, and Hank stuffed the operating

field with sponges to absorb the blood. Then they covered the wound with towels, lifted Luis up, and gently turned him over.

Fred began to perform external cardiac massage, laying his hands flat on Luis's chest, pushing downward, then releasing, and repeating the procedure.

An emergency team of physicians and nurses raced into the room, pushing in front of them a packed "crash cart," which contained a defibrillator, and drugs, among them epinephrine, which increases heartbeat.

"Hand me the eppie," the anesthesiologist urged.

He injected the drug straight into Luis's heart. At the same time, other anesthesiologists, who had come into the room with the crash team, went to work. One monitored the ventilator, another checked blood gases, while others pumped drugs through the various IVs that were already in place in Luis's body.

A nurse set the defibrillator unit to deliver voltage, then handed the attached paddles to Fred, who placed them on Luis's chest.

"Stand back." Then, "Hit it," Fred commanded.

The boy's arms and legs jerked convulsively as the current passed through his heart. The purpose of administering this countershock, called defibrillation, was to force all of the muscle cells to contract simultaneously, thereby restoring normal heart action.

Nothing happened with the first shock. Indeed, Luis now showed no cardiac activity at all, and the blood monitors pointed to another, related problem. He was suffering from acidosis, an abnormal reduction of alkalinity in the blood. It was probably the blood abnormality, complicated by instability in his autonomic system, which covers involuntary actions, that had caused the cardiac arrest.

Fred administered more countershocks—two, three, four, five. At this point, there were fifteen or more people crowded around the operating table, each performing like a member of a well-rehearsed drill team.

As the minutes ticked by, Fred mentally exhorted Luis: "Let's get it moving, old pal. Come on, come on."

Fred knew that the longer arrest persisted, the fewer chances there were that countershock would work. But it *had* to work. He hadn't come this far to lose Luis now, in this way.

Fred felt caught in a nightmare. He had at his disposal all the high technology in the world—scans, ultrasonic aspirator, operating scope, carbon dioxide laser, electrodes planted everywhere, and a damn defibrillator, too—and God knows, he wasn't doing any better than a native curer with a pile of herbs and bare hands. In fact, he was doing a lot worse.

But you were wrong, Mrs. Delgado, he thought, remembering that Carmen's mother had warned her the operation wouldn't work. Carmen *was* right to trust him. Fred unleashed all of his optimism, pushing it to the forefront of his mind. Of all his weapons, the one thing he could depend on most was his own innate drive to preserve life.

"The kid's coming around," one of the members of the emergency team said.

After thirty horrendous minutes, cardiac rhythm had finally been restored, followed by a return of blood pressure to normal levels. The restoration occurred so suddenly, it was almost difficult to believe there had been any crisis.

The members of the "crash team" gathered their equipment and departed, leaving everyone in the room utterly drained.

"Does this happen very often?" one of the medical students who was watching asked innocently.

There was an explosion of hysterical laughter, tinged with relief.

"If it did, would we all still be working here?" Fred asked.

He could remember only one similar incident, six years previously. As fate would have it, a television news team had been in the OR when it happened. The tapes were shown on local television that night, and the commentator explained that the surgery had been interrupted when the patient, a young man, developed "slight breathing difficulties." Fred couldn't imagine what the viewers must have thought when they saw him practically jumping up and down on the young man's chest—some breathing difficulties. Fortunately, the shots of the heart monitors, indicating imminent disaster, were never shown.

Now it was a comfort to hear those monitors beeping away normally, their mild fluctuations of sound as familiar to him as the gentle waves of the ocean would be to a navigator.

"Fred, are you thinking about closing?" the anesthesiologist asked.

Fred had thought about it, but only for a fleeting moment. If he terminated the procedure now, part of the tumor would be left in place, poised to renew its growth. With a malignant tumor you had to "reduce the oncologic burden," get out as much as possible, because every tiny bit left was a time bomb.

Unlike a benign tumor, there was no possibility that the remaining portions would wither away. He had to destroy the thing now, while it was at his mercy.

"We're going to continue with the surgery," Fred said.

The anesthesiologist's voice came loud and clear from behind the monitors, vehement in disapproval. There was the danger of another arrest, he argued.

Fred listened calmly, then countered with an argument of his own—completing the surgery was the only way to save this particular patient. Without removing all of the tumor this time, the prognosis was zero.

"I hope you know what the hell you're doing," the anesthesiologist grumbled.

"I do," Fred replied with great certainty.

Jeff said nothing. Fred had the feeling that if Jeff were in charge, he would have closed. He was generally less aggressive than Fred or more cautious, however you want to phrase it. It was a slight difference in style, but not in substance. Basically, their approach was the same—and this particular operation belonged to Fred. No matter how it came out, there wouldn't be any recriminations from Jeff. The only recriminations would be the ones in Fred's heart.

However, once Fred made a decision, he left all doubt behind.

"Let's turn him," he said to Jeff.

They put Luis on his stomach, and removed the sponges from the wound. Then Hank irrigated the wound with copious amounts of antibiotics. All of the manipulations during the arrest had significantly increased the danger of infection.

The operating microscope, which had been hastily moved out of the way, was brought back, and the surgery resumed its normal course.

Almost an hour later, the remainder of the tumor was gone. After giving one final burst, Fred turned off the Cavitron.

The going had been tough, because the swollen condition of the spinal cord made it difficult to avoid damaging normal tissue.

Fred was accustomed to the pain in his hands and shoulders at the end of these operations, rather like the way a ballet dancer becomes used to the agony of toe shoes. But today the pain was overwhelming—he felt as if every bone in his body had been stretched on the rack.

Jeff sutured the dura back together. Then the two surgeons replaced the backbone, attaching it with sutures that went through the bone. Three other sets of sutures were made to close the muscle, the fascia, and the skin. Finally, Hank placed a sterile dressing along the length of Luis's back, and Fred and Jeff turned the boy on his back.

The anesthesiologist removed the endotracheal tube, and Luis began to breathe normally. "You've got a guardian angel watching over you, Epstein," he said.

"No," Fred murmured, "Luis has."

By the time they got to the recovery room, taking along one of the medical students who spoke Spanish, Luis had regained consciousness.

He played the piggy game perfectly, moving his fingers and toes and then trying it again for effect, since he had received such a terrific response from the assembly.

But even though Luis understood the game well enough, there was still the possibility of brain damage. His arrest had lasted half an hour.

"Ask him what city he's in," Fred said.

"Nueva York," came back the answer.

"And who am I?"

When he understood Luis's reply, the medical student smiled.

"He says you are Dr. Epstein, the tall magician. And he wants to know where his teddy bear is."

Fred could have hugged Luis to pieces.

CHAPTER 16

FRED

What if I had lost Luis? I would have sat in my library long nights, barely talking to anyone, with my family knowing better than to try to talk to me. It would have been an agony. Still, I would have endured it, because it's the downside of what I do, and it has to be borne.

Neurosurgery has proved to be the most innovative aspect of neuroscience because its pioneers were able to undergo similar agonies. They were willing to joust with failure in order to expand the frontiers of knowledge.

At one point in his career, Sir Victor Horsley, the most important neurosurgeon of the nineteenth century, performed ten unsuccessful operations on pituitary tumors in a row. As he prepared to undertake the eleventh, a colleague warned him off, saying, "Victor, if you operate on that man, he will die."

"Of course he will," Horsley replied, "but if I don't operate, those who come after me will do no better."

Today, we're less arrogant than Sir Victor, more concerned, and rightly so, about the ethics of experimenting with patients' lives. Still, despite his seeming assurance, I don't know how Horsley could have borne all of those disasters. Maybe they were the reason he left surgery at the age of fifty to take up a second career as a social reformer.

The fact is that in neurosurgery—as perhaps in all of life— failure is just as important as success. I myself have brought failure to a high art, but I had a head start. Looking back, I think that doing poorly in school as a child may have been an advantage. I became persistent, and I learned not to mind being laughed at.

If the truth were told, the public would know that most new medical ideas prove to be completely or partially wrong. That's not important. What's important is to keep going, to keep churning out other approaches.

We need the courage to pursue new ideas and concepts, even if they don't pan out. Otherwise, our fear of being wrong keeps us from being right.

By some lucky break—genes, my parents, my stars—I'm not afraid of failing. In fact, I've learned to love my "mis-adventures" because, along with my successes, they're part of the evolving history of pediatric neurosurgery.

One of my favorite ideas is one I had in 1970 for arresting hydrocephalus. At that time, the CT scan did not exist, and magnetic resonance imaging was not even dreamed of. If any-one had predicted something like the MRI, he or she would have been laughed at and accused of talking science fiction.

Without scans to pick up signs of malfunctions early on, children with shunts were subject to significant complications, and even to death itself. Far better, I thought, to figure out how to stop the hydrocephalus without having the patient become shunt dependent.

A colleague and I discovered when we induced hydrocephalus in cats that the disease arrested itself naturally at a certain point. After being injected with kaolin, a drug that induces the accumulation of cerebrospinal fluid, the ventricles of the cats' brains expanded from one cc to three cc, then stabilized. All of the animals were acutely ill at first, but seventy-two hours later, they were free of hydrocephalus, and intracranial pressure had returned to normal.

What caused the "cure"? It was speculated that the ventricular surface had expanded to the point where it could absorb enough cerebrospinal fluid to achieve equilibrium.

It seemed that if we came up with some sort of "natural" shunting system for children, designed to mimic this physiological event, a permanent shunt might be avoided. We developed an "on-off shunt," which only drained fluid when a parent opened a valve for eight minutes, four times a day. If the fontanelle, the soft opening in the child's skull, ceased to bulge and the head didn't grow any larger, the use of the shunt was tapered off, then discontinued.

Approximately 20 percent of the children we treated in this manner became free of hydrocephalus and their intelligence developed normally. This was a great step forward. Although we clearly hadn't ironed out all the kinks, I was elated, convinced I had discovered the basis of the treatment of the future.

I felt so confident that I summarized our work at a professional meeting in 1973. Feeling terrific, I waited for the approbation of the group. But after my paper, a colleague, Howard Eisenberg, M.D., reported on research conducted with a Boston professor. Howard had also made cats hydrocephalic, but instead of suggesting that the fluid was absorbed through the expanded surface of the ventricles, he said that it drained through the central canal of the spinal cord. This was a pathway my fellow researcher and I had not thought of, and hearing about it really put a damper on my day.

Well, I thought, Howard and the professor must be misguided; *I* couldn't possibly be wrong.

I returned to the laboratory, eager to prove that I was correct. I thought all I had to do was to surgically obstruct the spinal cords of cats with arrested hydrocephalus. If the cats survived—and I was certain they would—it would show that the cerebrospinal fluid was being absorbed by the ventricular surface.

Each of the four cats I operated on died within six hours of surgery. Well, so much for being right.

I had every reason to feel embarrassed, but I've found that feeling bad is a waste of time. No idea that's well thought out can really be misguided, even if it turns out to be wrong, because we learn something from every investigation.

I had learned that hydrocephalus in cats could be arrested. At a certain point, as the intracranial pressure rises, the canal of the spinal cord becomes an alternative pathway for siphoning off fluid. Perhaps we could make that happen in humans by increasing intracranial pressure and forcing more fluid to be absorbed in the head.

At first, I simply wrapped the patients' heads with an Ace bandage, in a manner quite similar to a technique used in the nineteenth century. Then I developed an inflatable cap. We found that intracranial pressure increased at first, but later returned to normal levels, despite the maintenance of high pressure within the cap. Out of twenty children treated with this method, hydrocephalus was permanently arrested in ten.

A short time later, the CT scan was introduced, and many of the complications inherent in shunts have become history. With the advent of magnetic resonance imaging, we can follow these patients even more effectively. I no longer needed to try to control hydrocephalus by use of an inflatable cap.

However, Howard Eisenberg had shown that cerebrospinal fluid could accumulate in the central canal of the spinal cord. Could that knowledge have a usefulness for other central nervous system disorders? Spina bifida, for example.

Many infants born with spina bifida have a meningomyelocele—a protrusion of the lowest part of the spinal cord through a hole in the skin. I hypothesized that an accumulation of cerebrospinal fluid in the canal might have something to do with this protrusion. Perhaps the meningomyelocele developed, over time, in the mother's uterus as the fluid dissolved the lower end of the spinal cord.

I questioned more than two hundred mothers of children with a meningomyelocele, and all said they had experienced normal fetal movement until the last trimester of pregnancy; then movement had slowed down drastically. That, I thought, was when most of the damage occurred.

Could this damage be re-created in a laboratory animal by removing the bone overlying the abnormal spinal cord? I operated on several cats with dilated canals and found that it could.

So, by a convoluted route, I arrived at some understanding of how one facet of an embryological process might go wrong. Someday it may be possible to correct the problem, the dilation of the canal, surgically in utero, thus contributing to the prevention of meningomyelocele.

With each step we take in medical science, what's complex becomes clearer and, conversely, what seems fairly clear at the beginning can become more complex. One has to be able to live with this anomaly.

When I started operating on "inoperable" brainstem tumors in the early 1980s, not too much was known about these tumors, beyond their general classifications and location in a very tricky area.

The brainstem, which controls blood pressure, heartbeat, and breathing, forms the bottommost portion of the brain. It connects the cerebral hemispheres of the brain—the cerebrum and the cerebellum—with the spinal cord.

Despite its tiny size, the brainstem is the site of three important structures. The pons relays impulses between the cerebrum and the cerebellum and the spinal cord. The midbrain, a short portion of the brainstem between the pons and the cerebral hemispheres, relays the impulses that control body movements as well as other important functions. And the medulla oblongata controls breathing, heartbeat, swallowing, and numerous other functions.

For a long time, before the advent of MRI, there was no effort to be more descriptive about brainstem tumors, or to classify them according to their location, which might suggest operability. They were simply described as "inoperable."

But with the development of imaging techniques, we were able to identify three important subgroups of the gliomas that occur in the brainstem: diffuse, cervicomedullary, and focal. Diffuse tumors—tumors that have spread—are generally malignant gliomas of advanced grade. Cervicomedullary tumors—occuring at the junction of the medulla and the spinal cord—can be a "melting pot" of pathology, low grade or high grade, benign or malignant, but they are usually benign. Kevin Dagner and Roger Hendricks both had benign, low-grade cervicomedullary tumors, by far the most common variety in this subgroup. The third category, focal tumors, are located entirely within the medulla and are most often benign and of low grade.

Since cervicomedullary tumors and focal tumors are generally quite similar, we expected surgery on them to have the same results. But it didn't work out that way.

The first child I operated on for a focal tumor was Jonathan Morris, a four-year-old boy with a history of nausea, vomiting, impaired speech, and double vision. We were able to debulk 90 percent of the tumor, and microscopic pathology showed that it was a low-grade ganglioglioma.

In the recovery room, when we removed the breathing tube, Jonathan seemed to be fine; he was breathing on his own and in good spirits. I was delighted to give his parents the encouraging news.

But over the next twelve hours, bad things started to happen. Jonathan developed breathing difficulties and, a short time later, he went into respiratory arrest. The staff of the intensive care unit was able to revive him, but the arrest was followed by several episodes of aspiration pneumonia and neurological deterioration. Five weeks after surgery, Jonathan had lost his gag reflex and was unable to swallow. A feeding tube was inserted through a stab wound into his stomach, and though Jonathan is still alive, can walk and play, he is nevertheless dependent on the tube. Neurological symptoms remain, although the tumor has not returned.

We concluded that Jonathan's case was one of the inexplicable things that could happen in brainstem surgery, then in its formative stages.

However, over time, Jonathan's experience proved to be the norm for patients with focal tumors. We operated on six more such patients. In each case, the tumor was relatively easy to reach and debulk. Post-op, the patient did well until breathing problems developed, hours or days later, and the gag reflex became compromised. In some cases, a feeding tube or breathing tube, or both, was necessary. Although patients remained clinically stable afterward, their symptoms didn't change.

We couldn't figure out what was going wrong. In these operations, as in every operation we performed, evoked potentials and auditory responses had been monitored by electrodes. In none of these cases were there any significant changes during surgery, any delays in response time that would make us think that damage was being done.

As time went on, however, it became clear that there was something about the location of the tumor—in the medulla—that was causing our inability to pick up catastrophic results.

It took us some time to figure out that even though evoked potential readings during surgery might be normal in the medulla, they were apparently not a helpful measure of what was actually happening.

There was no way to get a good reading on the breathing center for this type of tumor. And by the time we discovered this, a number of patients had experienced surgery that may have been successful in curing the tumor, but had left permanent complications. Nowadays, we prevent these problems by leaving a breathing tube in place for three to four days after surgery on focal tumors.

The more I progress in my neurosurgical practice and in life, the more I see how everything is connected, failure to success, large to small. I was attracted to neurosurgery because I viewed the brain as a great, uncharted ocean, testing the bold venturer. It didn't take me long to learn that other central nervous system disorders, such as hydrocephalus, a far less "sexy" disorder for a neurosurgeon to grapple with, are also part of that great unknown, and that what we learn about one disorder is bound to have an effect on the others.

"What goes around, comes around," goes the old saying, meaning that what you give comes back to you, sometimes in an unexpected form. I have seen this happen time and time again, not only in medical science, but also with parents, who reach out to support other parents and find themselves strengthened in ways they hadn't thought possible.

Even in a child's death—perhaps the greatest failure in the cosmos—there can be gains, though there can never be compensation.

Five years after a favorite patient died, I was engaged in setting up a research fund for children with brain tumors. I wrote to his parents, who were quite well off financially, asking for their help.

They came to my office immediately, which meant they had to journey back to the same floor where their son had undergone physical therapy. And they had to see other children whose bodies and minds were ravaged by brain cancer and other diseases.

Everything these parents had experienced came rushing back, and the mother could barely make it to my office door. If they worked with me on this project, we would be in constant contact, and they would have to relive so much of what they were struggling to forget. Could these people risk getting reinvolved in that painful world? And if they did, would their efforts really make any difference?

But when the mother saw the other parents, the "newcomers," waiting to talk to me about their children, she realized that her own discomfort made no difference. She had to help.

"If anything you do produces any advance at all, my son's

passing won't have been totally without purpose," she said, wiping away tears.

Within months, the couple had established a research fund, and I had the wherewithal, first, to be able to pay for transportation and housing for patients and their families who could not otherwise afford to come to New York, and second, for the entire department—Jeff Allen, Jeff Wisoff, Rick Abbott, Tania Shaminski-Maher, and myself—to conduct research.

Now, it seems, we proceed by millimeters, in the same way the Cavitron destroys tumors, and sometimes we appear to be falling backward, but I know we're not. Bit by bit, survival rates have increased—and the gifts of time have been extended.

That couple's son, Frank Morella, Jr., Bonita Jeffers, Davy Feldman—they live on in some way in the lives of the children we have cured.

Last year, my son Jason came of bar mitzvah age. Many members of my family and a few close friends journeyed to Israel, where we had decided to hold the ceremony. It took place at Masada, the great fortress near the Dead Sea, where in 73 A.D., a lone band of Jewish defenders committed suicide, one by one, rather than surrender to the Roman invaders. Masada has become a symbol of Jewish resistance and nationalism, one of the most visited sites in the country.

As I proudly watched Jason read from the Torah, I remembered Davy Feldman's halting, indeed minimal, recitation from the same holy book. By some standards, it would have been thought a failure, by others a great triumph. Who was to decide?

It was possible that the very defenders of those ancient stones might have considered themselves failures, defeated, and unable to guess the inspiration they would provide for future generations.

The common denominator between Davy and the defenders was courage.

In medicine, as in everyday life, only courage counts if we are to move forward, because the meaning of the results—success or failure—can only be measured, and will surely *be* measured, by time.

CHAPTER 17

*T*he chapel of the funeral home was crowded when Fred arrived, late, for Sarah Glazer's funeral. Sarah was being buried, according to Jewish law, within twenty-four hours of her death, and that had given Fred little time to rearrange his schedule. He had hurried away from the hospital as soon as he could, leaving Rick Abbott to give a report to the parents of the patient they had just operated on.

He had looked around in vain for a seat and resigned himself to standing in the back, when he saw Lila Glazer signaling to him from the front row. She had saved a seat for him next to her.

Lila's appearance was strained but composed, in sharp contrast to the audible sobbing of some elderly people, apparently relatives, who sat in the row behind them.

Lila took Fred's hand. "I've cried all the tears I can cry for Sarah," she whispered.

He thought of those last days in the hospital, when Lila had wept copiously and Daniel had become strangely calm—an odd reversal of what he would have expected. But Fred no longer wondered at the way parents acted when they had to watch a child die. That duty has no equal in the devastation it produces, and anything short of suicide, Fred often thought, is acceptable behavior for a parent in this situation.

One mother's story was particularly heartbreaking. She was pregnant and close to the delivery of her second child when her five-year-old, Angela, became terminal.

"I want to have the baby here, at NYU, so I can be near Angie when she dies," the woman had pleaded.

She was on Medicaid, and scheduled to give birth at a city hospital. Fred offered to pay for an NYU delivery, but the obstetrician turned him down, saying he would absorb the cost himself.

Three days after the new baby was born, Angela died, while her mother held her hand.

The Glazers' final days with Sarah were not much different.

After it was decided that Sarah would receive no further treatment, she was moved to a quiet, private room, apart from the hustle and bustle of the unit, and cots were set up for Daniel and Lila.

They were with her round the clock, and Fred was often with them, offering support or just sitting quietly.

The obligations of a pediatric neurosurgeon, he believed, included a commitment to become part of a distraught family in its hour of need. It was a painful experience—and one that he often felt like running away from—but he knew there was no way to separate himself from the family's emotional turbulence. In fact, he could help them best by becoming a part of it.

There were others who joined in this sharing—Tania, Rick, Jeff Wisoff, and the nurses on the unit, who shielded Daniel and Lila from outside intrusion as much as possible, and themselves from the constant calls of relatives.

"Every minute I spend talking with you is a minute I could be with the family," Fred heard a nurse say in a kindly fashion to a cousin of Daniel's.

Among the last questions Sarah had typed when she could still use her computer were these: "What will happen when I die?" "Will it hurt?"

Daniel explained that he didn't know what would happen exactly, but he knew that Sarah would be in a good place and that she would be at peace. No, he said emphatically, it wouldn't hurt to die.

The doctors and nurses tried to make that last promise a reality. Sarah was given sedatives to help her sleep and large doses of morphine administered intravenously for the pain. The mechanical apparatus that interfered with her comfort, the other IVs and the feeding tube, were removed. The only equipment that remained was a nasal cannula, a tube to supply oxygen, which made her breathing less labored.

One by one, her systems shut down, and she became semi-comatose. She looked as fragile as a newborn baby. Lila lay in bed with Sarah, holding her in her arms, almost as if she were nursing her. The sheet was wet with Lila's tears.

Daniel sat in a corner, looking through a pile of Sarah's old photographs. He had little to say, not even to Fred, whom he had plied with questions for so many years. Now the questioning had come to an end.

Sarah died in Lila's arms one night when Fred was in the room, shortly after Tania had paid a visit.

"She was waiting for the two of you to say good-bye," Lila said in an odd voice.

Then a nurse took Sarah's body from her, and Lila became convulsed with sobs.

"I have no life now, I have no life," she kept repeating,

forgetting about Daniel and her other daughter, Naomi. Sarah had been Lila's "work," almost her entire existence, for eleven years.

Now, at the funeral, Fred shared yet another glimpse of what Lila's world had been like.

"Do you see that woman?" she said, glancing across the room.

The woman was a pharmaceutical company representative, someone who had worked with Lila in supplying the drugs Sarah needed at home. Two of Sarah's home health nurses were in the chapel, too.

"I'm going to miss these people," Lila said. "They know more about what I've been through than the friends I've had all my life."

The rabbi who was conducting the service, a colleague of Daniel's, was talking about what an angel Sarah had been.

Angelic? Fred didn't remember her that way. She had always been feisty, even as an infant after her first surgery, when she had glared up at him from beneath a bandage twice the size of her head, as though challenging him to help her fight. Tough and enduring, those were better words for this kid. Sarah had worked hard for every breath of life, and used them to the best advantage.

Fred felt that strange sensation one gets when being stared at from behind. He turned around and saw several pairs of eyes fixed on him, the owners wondering, no doubt, why he was seated with the family.

Perhaps the starers deduced that he was that doctor the Glazers talked about so much, the one who had extended Sarah's life when everyone expected her to die.

In the Glazer family, Fred knew, he was touted as a "miracle worker." But if there had been any "miracle" at all, it belonged first to Sarah and her family and then to modern technology—

and even more, to history. Without the long, painful record of trial and error that produced modern neurosurgery, he would have had nothing to offer Sarah.

How to relieve the horror of intractable head pain—that question was as old as mankind itself, and the answer had been slow in coming.

Attempts to find an answer went back very far in history, even to Neolithic times, when cavemen carved holes in the skull with sharpened rocks or pointed pieces of flint, perhaps with the intention of relieving pressure. We know that some of the "patients" lived, because remains of heads have been discovered with smooth holes in them, showing that the wounds had time to heal.

Fred had always wondered how the prehistoric "curers" knew where to drill or by what means? Did they think there was a "spirit" growing inside the head? The answers were hidden in the dawn of time, yet Fred felt there must have been some kind of drive at work there, the same one he felt himself, to get at a hidden monster and force its evacuation.

In ancient times, the brain's anatomy began to be better understood. In 400 B.C., Hippocrates, the father of medicine, suggested that a patient with a head injury could be helped by trephining, known today as a craniectomy, the removal of a section of the skull. There was no attempt, though, at penetrating the brain itself and removing a tumor, because tumors were not known to exist. Later on, when brain tumors did become recognized, they were thought to be inoperable. It wasn't until the nineteenth century that the picture changed.

Then improvements in anesthesia and increased understanding of the circulatory system and physiology made "brain surgery" possible for the first time.

Even so, few had the courage to venture into that murky region.

A major pioneer was that same Sir Victor Horsley who had performed so many unsuccessful operations for pituitary tumors. Horsley was a hard-driving Englishman, an accomplished surgeon by the age of twenty-nine and an indefatigable researcher. By inserting a balloon into an animal's brain, for example, he showed that a growing brain tumor could press against the skull and cause damage. Then, by deflating the balloon, he demonstrated how the brain could resume its normal function once the "tumor" was eliminated. Horsley conducted experiments on hundreds of animals, accumulating the greatest understanding of the brain up to that point.

In 1886, he performed ten brain operations on human beings, thereby toppling the barriers against brain surgery. It was like opening up a floodgate. Over the next decade, hundreds of surgeons published accounts of brain surgeries they had performed.

But despite the daring of the Victorian neurosurgeons— Horsley was knighted by the queen for his achievements— brain tumor operations were so often fatal that the British Medical Society considered forbidding them.

Fred shuddered to think of how Sarah and his other patients would have fared during that time. There was so little chance of an adult's surviving, the death of a child was a foregone conclusion. Almost nothing was known of the physiological differences between children and adults, but it wouldn't have mattered. The diagnostic and surgical methods needed to save lives weren't there in any case.

The situation improved considerably as a result of the efforts of the next great pioneer, Harvey Cushing. In the early 1900s, Cushing decided to become the first American brain surgeon, wondering, as he did so, why he was interested in a specialty where the surgery killed one out of every two to three patients. Perhaps, Fred speculated, it was because Cushing was determined to change things—a mind-set with which Fred identified.

Cushing realized that successful surgery depended on choosing the right tumors and operating early rather than after a case became nearly "hopeless," as was then the practice. He also recognized the importance of standardizing and refining technique—these advances would greatly increase the amount of time devoted to a brain tumor operation—and of monitoring the patient's blood pressure and cardiac rate during surgery. This led to substantial improvements in survival rates.

In 1910, Cushing's accomplishments got wide publicity when he operated on Major General Leonard Wood, a national hero of the Spanish-American War. Wood, himself a physician, suffered from a type of tumor that Cushing had been studying for ten years, a meningioma. But Cushing had never removed a meningioma that, like Wood's, extended beyond the tissue covering the brain and into the organ itself.

Cushing hesitated to operate, but Wood demanded the surgery, saying that he was no longer able to climb a ladder in front of his men and that it was growing increasingly difficult to conceal the nature of his illness.

Eleven days after the surgery, the paralysis in Wood's left leg was gone and so were the seizures he had been suffering. "I owe everything to you," he wrote to Cushing, shortly after he was sworn in as army chief of staff.

By 1930, thanks in large measure to Cushing's skill and the vast amount of research he had done, the mortality rate for brain surgery he performed had fallen to 5 percent. Cushing had advanced neurosurgery so considerably, he could almost be said to have invented it.

He even marked the inauguration of the high-tech era, Fred

thought, having been the first to use an "electric knife" to cut tissue and cauterize bleeding.

Suppose, Fred mused, that Sarah had been under Cushing's care, in the hands of the great Boston Brahmin himself, with his tireless methodology and perfectionistic drive to excel. Even Cushing could not have given Sarah the life span that Fred and his associates had provided.

For time, a *real* gift of time, one had to thank the adjuvant therapies and technological advances of the late twentieth century. Take the operating microscope, for example.

Although some forms of microscope had been used in operating rooms since the 1920s, it was not until 1953 that an instrument was designed that had two eyepieces, a camera hookup, a video monitor, and its own source of light. Although some surgeons used the scope as early as the 1960s, it came into routine use only about seventeen years ago. With the operating microscope, Fred could spot and cauterize blood vessels that were no thicker than a human hair.

Then there were the CT scan, introduced in the early 1970s, and the MRI, in the mid-1980s. And the laser, and the Cavitron.

These were the underpinnings of Sarah Glazer's fragile, and bountiful, eleven years.

We'll do better in the future, Sarah, Fred promised, I swear we will. In the vast cosmos of the brain, we're only at the beginning of discovery, in prehistory, really. It was not quite one hundred years ago that Sir Victor Horsley performed those first tentative brain operations, and less than a century since Harvey Cushing made brain surgery successful.

Someday, Fred was certain, there would be no need for ceremonies like this one, eulogizing a young life vanquished by a brain tumor.

Fred noticed that Daniel had ascended the pulpit, carrying

with him a pile of Sarah's computer printouts. He had to compose himself several times before he attempted to speak.

Daniel had a great deal to share with the mourners.

"I want to tell you about the good times in my daughter's life," he began, "and there were many, because Sarah gobbled up life in great bites.

"She loved the sky. She used to wake up at three o'clock in the morning, wake up Lila and me, and say, 'Let's count the stars.' When we shooed her out, pleading for another hour of sleep, she would leave our room dramatically, saying she would do it herself. The thing about Sarah was that she could do that. She knew how to be alone in the night.

"There were many other things Sarah loved to do. One was poring over maps. She could tell you where every important capital in the world was and every challenging mountain range. She planned to visit these famous sites sometime.

"Instead, she had to watch videos. After viewing a nature video one day, she wrote on her computer, 'Old Faithful is my favorite geyser. It has a mind of its own, like me. It knows when to say "hello" and when to go away.'

"Sarah loved to walk with me in the park near our home, recording the birds we saw in a book her sister bought for her. Some days, she could walk for an hour without stopping. Those were wonderful days. She loved to ride her bike, too, and we really were proud when she could finally make it, as she said, 'around the whole, entire block.'

"She was a reader, too, and she loved to be in school. But she couldn't always go there, because she was often in her other home, New York University Medical Center. With each admission, she was greeted by a group of familiar nurses and aides. To them, Sarah was, 'Miss Miraculous,' but she was often ambivalent about this second home. She wrote, 'I feel glad to see the nurses. I don't feel glad to see the nurses. I wish they would stop giving me shots. There's nothing else to say.'

"Sarah knew that she was very sick, but she planned for the future, nonetheless. 'In a few years, I will have a career,' she wrote. 'I will be a rabbi in New York City, or maybe at Disney World.'

"When I told her that there probably weren't any rabbis at Disney World, she gave me the most incredulous look. 'That's dumb,' she snapped, using one of her favorite expressions. And the steeliness in her eyes confirmed her determination. I knew what she was thinking. She would be the first to do this fantastic thing, to become a rabbi at Disney World. I've grown very fond of this cockeyed notion."

Fred smiled. Hearing Daniel talk about Sarah's life in such a positive way brought back happy memories of his own.

He remembered the day of the monkeys, three years ago.

The day had begun with Fred's receiving a call from a doctor in a small town in Connecticut.

"Dr. Epstein? I've got two infants here, twins, and I think they may be hydrocephalic. Can you check them out for me?"

Within hours the "patients" had arrived, twin chimpanzees. The caller had been a veterinarian who apparently thought Fred would deduce the nature of the infants from the name of the institution he gave, a recognized animal hospital. But he had reckoned without Fred's notorious capacity for overlooking names.

The chimps were installed in Jeff Wisoff's office—Jeff was out of town—where they were examined and found to be normal. But then they had to wait to be picked up. It was all JoAnn Baldwin could do to keep them away from the piles of Jeff's possessions, which revealed so much of his scholarly personality: reprints of recently published academic papers, lists of notes on those papers, and cherished photographs of his wife and two daughters.

In the meantime, Fred's waiting area was filled with human patients, including Sarah.

Every so often, loud-pitched squeals and squeaks emitted from Jeff's office.

"What's that?" a parent asked.

"Just a pair of . . . of infant twins," Fred explained.

JoAnn slipped in and out of Jeff's office in an effort to keep the chimps quiet, trying to be as unobtrusive as possible.

But the noises continued, even as everyone pretended to be unaware of them. Everyone, that is, but eight-year-old Sarah.

"Babies? That's dumb," she said.

Slipping off Daniel's lap, she marched up to the door of the office and pushed it open, revealing the truth to all as vividly as the child in the story of the emperor's new clothes.

"Monkeys!" Sarah exclaimed. "Are you making them better, too?"

"There's nothing wrong with them," Fred said.

He let Sarah cuddle one of the animals, savoring the joy in her eyes as she held the little furry body against her own.

"She loves the zoo," Daniel whispered, and once again, Fred realized the value of the time he had been able to give to Sarah. Hers was far from a wasted life. Despite her pain, she experienced great happiness, and gave it back in abundance to those around her.

Sarah and Daniel played with the monkeys until it was time for Fred to examine her.

"Thanks," Daniel said when they left an hour or so later. "You made our day."

After their departure, Fred felt good for a long time, just

as he did now at her funeral. It was an odd sensation, but somehow he didn't find it incongruous. In a strange way, Sarah's funeral had turned into an upbeat occurrence.

Fred realized that Daniel had resolved to celebrate rather than mourn Sarah's life, to value her time on earth instead of dwelling on its limited nature. In Sarah's death, Daniel had apparently found the meaning for which he had vainly searched while she was alive.

Daniel's voice was calm and melodious, his eyes glowing with a kind of fire. His last words to the congregants concerned Fred. "Sarah's story is also the story of her doctor, Fred Epstein," he said, "and Fred's stubborn faith that Sarah might live to grow up. Last night, I phoned Fred and asked him to say a few words here today."

Fred ascended the pulpit and put his arms around the man who had become as much a brother as his own siblings, Simon and Abram. He could feel the moisture on Daniel's face, perspiration mixed with some tears. Some of the wetness fell on Fred's own cheek, and he didn't bother to brush it away.

As Fred assembled his thoughts, his eyes glanced down at the pile of computer printouts, which Daniel had left behind. I'm looking at Sarah's life, he thought. Then, just like Daniel, he understood how to express that life best.

"I want to tell you a story," he said, looking straight at the assembly, "about a feisty little girl and a pair of baby monkeys."

CHAPTER 18

In February, a few weeks after Sarah Glazer's funeral, winter set in with a vengeance and with it, an upsurge in the caseload of patients—ten with brain tumors, five with spinal cord tumors—and a seemingly endless round of complex problems, including congenital skull and spinal disorders, shunt insertions, and revisions, procedures to correct problems with a shunt.

On Valentine's Day, Fred and Kathy, along with Jeff Wisoff and his wife, Debbie, attended a wedding in Brooklyn.

The bride and groom, Alice and Tom, had both been hydrocephalics since birth and between them, had undergone almost 150 shunt operations.

Four days before the wedding, Tom had showed up at the hospital with a blinding headache, and an emergency surgery was performed on the shunt.

Afterward, Fred asked Tom, "Have you thought about postponing the wedding?"

"No way," Tom replied. "Not with what we'd have to pay the caterer. Besides, what's a little surgery to someone like me?"

The ceremony went on as planned. At the church, Fred and Jeff kept their eyes glued to the groom's back. Each time he swayed ever so slightly, the two physicians looked at each other, wondering whether they would have to cart him off to the hospital.

But except for those wobbly moments, the ceremony went off without a hitch.

Later, in the reception hall, Fred stood up and applauded along with the other guests as the caterer introduced "for the first time as man and wife, Mr. and Mrs. Thomas O'Flaherty."

When the music began, Fred and Kathy danced together, dance after dance.

"There's something magical about this reception," Kathy murmured, snuggling her head against his shoulder.

"Yes," Fred grinned. "I got here on time."

But he knew what she meant. The trappings were familiar enough for a large wedding—groaning tables of food, lively music, and happy relatives lifting glass after glass of champagne—yet the atmosphere in the room went beyond mere merrymaking. Amid it all, there was an air of thanksgiving, as if the whole event were a special gift.

Which it was. Until very recently, a wedding like this one would have been inconceivable. The bride and groom would not have lived to grow up, much less marry, and plan on having a family, as Tom had confided to Fred they intended to do.

For Fred, dancing at that wedding was like being in a dream. In his arms he held the person who was dearest to him in the world; all about him there were sounds of joy, joy that was due, at least in part, to his efforts and to Jeff's. He felt totally loved by everyone in the room, and feeling that way filled a very deep need.

Fred may have imagined it, but spring seemed to follow

quickly on the heels of the O'Flaherty wedding. The city seemed lighter, bathed in an illusion of rebirth, the way it looked each year at this time. In the Epstein apartment, there was a new acquisition, the tapestry of Fred's dog, Chloe, walking her master. With Sarah's death, Lila Glazer wrote, she had been able to complete it.

The parade of patients and parents in and out of Fred's office continued. In a spurt of spring cleaning, JoAnn Baldwin sorted through all of the file drawers, removing old records that could be more conveniently stored elsewhere. Fred tried to straighten out his desk, which was a pretty strange turn of events.

Some other strange things happened, too.

Early one evening, Fred was checking on a patient who, the nurses said, had been nearly comatose for several hours. Absentmindedly, he picked up a cookie from an almost empty box on the night table.

As Fred walked down the hall, savoring the last crumb, he heard the voice of the supposedly unresponsive child cry loudly, "Dr. Epstein took my last cookie." He raced back to the room along with a nurse, to find the patient sitting up in bed, totally coherent and demanding a new box of goodies.

A few days later, another oddity occurred. A physician from a European university arrived on a three-month fellowship, having planned for some time, he said, to do research on a new type of shunting procedure. When Fred agreed to provide space and laboratory animals, the doctor looked disappointed.

"Laboratory animals?" he asked. "Don't you have an extra patient you can let me have?"

Just as Fred wondered whether he had heard correctly, the man repeated the request. Fred turned him down of course, but for the next few weeks, he watched the doctor carefully, as if Count Dracula had managed to join his staff.

By the time he felt more comfortable with the physician, early summer had arrived, and with it—it turned out—one week that contained two pieces of good news.

First, Alice O'Flaherty stopped by after a visit to her gynecologist and announced that she was pregnant.

Then a letter came from Ashley, Mississippi. Inside was a newspaper clipping about Kevin Dagner's remarkable recovery, and a note from Ina Bea.

"Dear Dr. Epstein," Ina Bea had started to write, then crossed out the words "Dr. Epstein," and replaced them with "Fred."

"Last week," the letter went on, "there was a brief spot on a cable channel about the work you do—if only we'd seen such a program when Kevin was so desperately ill—and I decided a thank-you was long overdue. As I watched the program, I began to relive that emotional week last November when you worked on Kevin's brainstem tumor. There was one scene where you were speaking to a worried mother as her daughter was about to go into surgery. Her anxiety was so evident that I found myself fighting back tears, as I remembered how scared I was when Kevin was the patient. One thing that kept me going was your reassuring confidence.

"Dr. Sparks says that Kevin is doing well. He's healthy and active, and right now, he's attending a summer camp with a good soccer program. He asked me to tell you that he's had more 'saves' than anyone else in the goalie position. He says you'll want to know about that."

Fred smiled, remembering how Kevin had had to struggle to learn to walk again. Kevin had told him all about it, and Fred himself had played a part.

The struggle had begun three days after surgery, when a slender black woman, carrying a tote bag and a red balloon, sat down near his bed.

"Kevin," she said, smiling at him, "my name is Darryl Benson. I'm a physical therapist, and I'm going to help you start moving around."

Kevin stirred eagerly. Moving around was just what he wanted to do. It seemed as if he'd been in bed forever.

Darryl held out the balloon.

"Let me see you touch it with your right hand," she said. "That's good. And now your left."

Kevin's left arm was bent at the elbow, and his hand seemed to be stuck to his side. It was quite an effort to free it and make a feeble lunge at the balloon. Kevin felt embarrassed.

"That's all right," Darryl said, touching the hand softly.

He heard her explain to his mother that Kevin was suffering from too much "tone," or tension, in his muscles, and that the tone would decrease as the swelling in his brain went down.

Darryl placed a pillow under Kevin's left armpit to raise his arm, then showed Ina Bea how to help him extend the arm and keep it straight.

From the tote bag, she withdrew a set of four blocks, and asked Kevin to stack them with his left hand, one on top of the other.

"Keep practicing," Darryl called out as she left the room. "You'll get there."

A few days later, she was back with a wheelchair and whisked Kevin down to the fifth floor of the Rusk Institute, to the rehabilitation unit near Fred's office.

Before he could try to walk, Kevin had to learn basic movements all over again: getting up on his hands and knees, raising himself on an elbow, sitting up without losing his balance, and, hardest of all, rolling over in one fluid motion. At Darryl's direction, he practiced the rollovers on a "mat table," a thick pad supported by an iron frame.

He was gyrating madly, trying to get his legs to follow the rest of his body, when Fred entered the room.

Fred checked on all his patients when they were in rehab, cheering them on as a parent would do, because the unit was too crowded to permit the real parents to be present.

"I feel like a baby on this mat," Kevin whispered to Fred. "I want to walk."

"You will, pal, you will," Fred reassured him.

The next day, Fred walked out of his office and encountered Kevin, preparing to walk with the aid of the parallel bars in the hallway.

Darryl had placed a thick canvas belt, called a "gait belt," around his waist so that she could support him in the middle of his body without interfering with his movement.

Though Kevin's left arm had become more relaxed, his whole left side was still quite weak, and he leaned heavily on his right leg. Darryl confided to Fred that Kevin, like most patients, had virtually no idea of what his body was doing. He thought he was walking straight.

Darryl stood Kevin in front of a mirror, so that he could learn to monitor his body.

"Think about where your nose is," she said, "and your belly button. Try to find the center of your body."

Kevin concentrated hard and as he did so, he stood up straighter.

As Kevin walked along the hall, Darryl continued to urge him on: "Pull your leg through, straighten your knee, tuck in your hip. You've done it in the mirror. You can do it now." Occasionally, she'd hold his leg straight, so he could get a sense of what it felt like that way.

Physically, it was tough going, and mentally it was even tougher. The hallway was crowded with children, some a whole lot younger than Kevin, who seemed to be doing better

236

than he was. On the bars in front of him, a small girl moved along swiftly.

Perspiration dripped from Kevin's face. Suddenly he stopped and pushed away Darryl's hand.

"I'm tired. I quit," he said, barely holding back tears.

Fred tried to keep from showing the sympathy he felt, sympathy which wouldn't do Kevin any good.

"Hey there," he said, determined to be firm. "You're an athlete, Kevin. You've got to get back into condition."

"I'll wait till I get home," Kevin murmured.

"It'll be a lot harder then," Fred insisted.

Kevin looked so sad. It had been centuries, Fred reflected, since he'd been a carefree little boy. Kevin needed some fun.

That evening, after rounds were finished, Fred wheeled Kevin back down to rehabilitation. He and Kevin watched as a group of Rusk Institute patients, occupying wheelchairs, lined up their "vehicles" at the end of the hall. They were preparing to race one another, a favorite sport on some evenings. Other patients stood around, some supported by canes or walkers, waiting for the event to begin.

When it did, Kevin was amazed by the speed and agility with which the wheelchairs zigzagged down the corridor, the occupants manipulating them in race after race as skillfully as if they were in the Indy 500. Each contestant had his or her partisans, and Kevin, Fred observed, was soon rooting for a boy who seemed to be close to his own age.

"I don't think I could do what he's doing," Kevin commented ruefully.

"Fortunately, you won't have to," Fred tossed back. "You won't be in a wheelchair very long. That boy will never be out of one."

Kevin looked at him somberly. "I guess you mean I'm pretty lucky," he said.

After that, Kevin worked like a demon, and by the time he left the hospital several weeks later, his balance was greatly improved.

Fred hugged him good-bye.

"I'm so proud of you, buddy," he said.

Kevin hesitated before getting into the taxicab. A nurse had told him, he said finally, that Fred gave each discharged patient four tickets, and box seats at that, to a Yankee game.

"Sure, that's true," Fred replied. "And I would have given them to you. But your folks are taking you straight home."

"Well," Kevin answered, "save some tickets for me. I may be back someday. I mean, on vacation or something."

Fred had smiled at the thought of Ina Bea's choosing to visit New York of her own free will, and he hoped she would never again have to visit it any other way.

Now, eight months later, it looked as if his hopes for Kevin were coming true. The tumor showed no sign of recurrence, and the boy had resumed a normal life, right down to playing a terrific soccer game. In Fred Epstein's pantheon of news, there was none better, unless it was something that bordered on the miraculous, like what had happened to Luis Olmedo.

Four days after Luis's surgery, Fred received a written report from Doug Miller, the neuropathologist.

"Received in formalin are two specimens," it began in typical fashion. "The first one is labeled 'spinal cord tumor' and the second, 'Cavitron aspirate.' "

The tumor cells, the report went on to say, were a mixture of malignant and benign cells, with the benign cells predominating.

After the first operation three years previously, the pathologist had determined that all of Luis's tumor consisted of malignant astrocyte cells. But with the development of more sophisticated staining techniques since the first surgery, it was possible to see cells that couldn't be distinguished before—the neuronal or nerve cells—and these were benign.

So, Luis's tumor was mixed rather than totally malignant, and the really good news was that such tumors usually took a longer time to recur or might never recur. That made Luis's outlook much more favorable than it had been, particularly since an MRI, taken a few days after the surgery, showed no trace of residual tumor.

The killer was completely gone—and it might not be coming back. And to think that he almost hadn't operated, had almost let Luis go home with the tumor eating up his spine, poised to paralyze and then kill.

Fred thanked the something deep within himself, a drive so deeply ingrained that he didn't even have to identify it as faith, that had pressed him to carry on.

Then he hurried to Nine East to give the good news to Carmen and Jorge Olmedo.

When he told Lourdes Suarez what to say to them, her eyes filled with tears of joy.

"Oh Fred, I'm so glad," Lourdes breathed, and he realized that she, a nurse who had seen too many children die, was as grateful as he was for every piece of good news.

In precise Spanish, Lourdes told the Olmedos about the revised diagnosis of Luis's tumor, and the fact that no follow-up chemotherapy or radiation would be necessary.

Carmen and Jorge looked at each other with relief. They began an excited conversation in Spanish, which ended with Jorge taking Carmen in his arms.

She drew back from him, embarrassed in front of the doctor and nurse.

"Will it come back again?" Carmen asked.

"I hope not," Fred replied, stressing the positive, as was his habit.

"I should not have asked," Carmen said, crossing herself. "It is sufficient, what has happened."

Carmen's statement made Fred feel closer to her than he ever had before. Its wisdom banished the gap between the caring, seeking person she was and the reserved pose she presented to the world.

He had, at last, managed to enter the mind that was so different from his own, yet very much the same.

Carmen's statement, too, helped him resolve a conflict he had been grappling with for several days, one that concerned another parent.

Elizabeth Buchanan had brought her son Richard to see him, carrying with her an MRI, performed at another medical center, that showed a brainstem tumor. She had come to Fred, Mrs. Buchanan said, because he was reputed to be "the best," and, she didn't need to add, she was accustomed to having the best.

Fred explained the risks of the surgery, as he did with all parents, and ended by saying, in an optimistic tone, that he thought he could make Richard well.

She didn't respond to his encouraging smile, or to his exhortation that they would need to work together. She refused to acknowledge that they were at the beginning of a challenging process; she wanted answers.

"You *think* you can make Richard well?" Mrs. Buchanan questioned. The tone reminded him of his mother's query, "Have you done your best, your *very* best?"—and its implication that he was failing in some way.

His mother had only wanted the best for her child, too, but brain surgery was another sphere where there were no exact answers, just hope, skill, and courage, rooted in the belief that one could make a difference.

It didn't get any more definitive than that; yet Mrs. Buchanan seemed to be demanding a guarantee.

Everything about her spelled trouble, Fred thought. She was a malpractice suit waiting to happen, one of the few parents who failed to tap his usual feeling of sympathy.

He had just about decided not to take the case, when his experience with Carmen Olmedo made him realize that he never really knew what was inside a parent's heart until he worked with him or her. Comparing the two women—one used to having nothing, the other to having everything—he wondered if they were so different after all. There was a commonality to having a child with a life-threatening illness that went beyond wealth, class, nationality.

There was also a mandate for helping such a child that went beyond a doctor's own puny desire to protect himself from trouble.

Fred saw the crevices wrought by pain on Richard Buchanan's young face; those crevices had no business being there. He saw the potential for extending the boy's life.

And he remembered what Jeff Allen had said to him years ago, after they had met with one frightened family to discuss treatment options. "You know, Fred, it's really a privilege to be allowed into people's lives at a time like this."

A privilege. That was it.

He would tell Rochelle Sedita, the office staffer in charge of scheduling, to put Richard Buchanan on the operating schedule. He would make rounds. Then he would go home and hug his own children.

It was sufficient.

CHAPTER 19

Midsummer. The hot prairie sun beat down on the small suburban housing development, keeping the occupants of the split-level structures locked inside their air-conditioned quarters.

The enforced captivity seemed to make Marnie's condition worse, Grace Brinn thought, or maybe it only seemed that way.

She had to admit that her eight-month-old daughter had been acting funny for weeks, since before the heat wave set in.

An active, appealing infant, Marnie had suddenly changed. "It's as if all the zip has gone out of her," Grace complained to her husband. She was right. Now all Marnie did was lie on her back, staring up at her mother and father, not responding to their coos or chatter. If they tried to sit her up, she'd fall over.

Feeding time, once a happy opportunity to communicate with the baby, had become a nightmare, since Marnie rapidly vomited back in a projectile fashion most of what she ate.

And she was clearly in discomfort, whimpering frequently,

and the past week or so, she'd been pulling on her left ear, as though she were attacking some pain.

The doctor found no ear infection or any other indication of infection. Marnie wasn't running a fever, he pointed out.

Perhaps the vomiting and the lethargy pointed to some sort of food allergy. He would arrange for testing, but in the meantime he suggested certain dietary changes.

The allergy idea struck Grace as wrong. But she kept quiet. She was a young, first-time mother with a full-time job and a cranky infant on her hands. In one month, she had gone from being a parent who rarely called the doctor, to one who called him three times a day. She felt guilty. Everyone, her husband, her mother-in-law, and even the doctor, seemed to imply that she was doing something wrong even by asking for help.

"What *is* it, Mrs. Brinn?" the physician asked recently, when she finally got through to him.

"Marnie's balance is off. I sit her up, and she topples over," Grace said.

"It takes some babies longer than others to sit up. Perhaps you're forcing her," the doctor said.

"She's been sitting up for months."

"Well, maybe it's one of those viruses that's not accompanied by a fever. Let's give it some time to clear up. Remember, a child will respond to your anxiety, so try to relax," and the doctor concluded the conversation.

She was tired of being patronized. She was tired of being scared. Something was very wrong with Marnie, and Grace Brinn didn't know what to do next.

CHAPTER 20

FRED

I never thought that my office could become more hectic than it usually is, but that August, it did. We learned, on relatively short notice, that we would be moving out of suite 518 into more spacious quarters, so we set to work planning and packing.

As summer drew to a close, there were boxes everywhere, each one labeled by JoAnn Baldwin as to its contents and destination. Small piles of debris lay scattered about on the carpeting, and the pictures and photographs that made my office so familiar and comfortable were gone, buried somewhere in one of the endless boxes.

My surroundings were denuded, and growing more bare by the minute. I had the uneasy feeling, as I listened to the sounds of the packing all around me, that both my desk and desk chair could be snatched away from me at any moment, even as I sat there working.

Amid the chaos, our work continued as usual. There was no respite from the ringing phones, the pink PLEASE

CALL reminder slips—and the worried parents. I would need to see them, even if I had to ask them to sit on packing crates.

One of the parents who arrived at this time was Grace Brinn.

When Natalie Cutrone brought her into my office, I thought at first that she might be an adolescent patient, that's how young she looked, just about the age of my daughter Samara, who is a college student.

She looked like Samara, too, blond hair, pug nose, and gray eyes. But unlike Samara, Grace was carrying the burden of having a critically ill child. And when I looked into her eyes, I could no longer mistake them for those of an adolescent. There was no trace of youth in eyes that had grown old in such a short amount of time.

Grace spoke in a soft voice, barely a whisper.

She stared at the nineteenth-century quilt, the only object left hanging on the wall. She seemed unable to express her response to it, but it was clear that at some level the quilt gave her pleasure.

I remembered how Ina Bea Dagner had enjoyed the quilt when I first met her in the fall. And as I listened to Grace Brinn's story, I couldn't help reflecting on how similar it was to Ina Bea's.

Grace said she had kept "bothering" her doctor about Marnie's symptoms until, at last, he agreed to have an MRI performed. The MRI showed that the baby was suffering from a fast-growing tumor of the cerebellum, a type of tumor that tends to metastasize rapidly along the brain and the spinal cord, through the cerebrospinal fluid.

"When I heard that, it was like I wanted to die," Grace murmured.

"I know," I said.

She looked at me, the gray eyes misting over, and for a second I could see the teenager inside.

The doctor referred Grace to a surgeon affiliated with the local hospital who told her that the tumor was inoperable. The infant was too young for surgery and the tumor too advanced to be treated in any other way. Marnie, he said, had only a few months to live.

"I couldn't handle it, I just couldn't," Grace told me. "And it made me crazy when my mother-in-law told me I could have another baby soon. It was like she expected me to throw Marnie away."

Grace was angry at everyone—the doctor, her husband, her mother-in-law and, particularly, herself.

She wasn't capable of expressing the guilt she felt, nor was she prepared to give Marnie up, even when her minister advised her to accept what seemed to be the will of God.

"It felt like I was burning in hell," Grace told me, "but the worst thing was that I was there all alone."

Grace's experience was not new to me. I'd heard it many times before. But there, in the empty stillness of the room, her words had a special clarity, as if we were getting down to the essence of the thing. The room became filled with the intensity of her emotions, and I could feel myself responding to them.

No parent should have to go through this, I thought. My anger rose, as it had the previous week when I first learned of Grace's situation through a letter she sent me.

She had heard about me, she said, from a friend who saw a clip on a television program, and she hoped I would excuse her poor spelling.

"I'm desperated for your help," Grace pleaded. "I know that your not God, but I just want a second opinion from you. My daughter is so wonderful, and she is the only child that I have, and I love her so much. I'm just not satisfy with these doctors out here. As I come to close my letter, I pray that you will answer me soon." And she noted her home number and the number of the restaurant where she worked as a waitress.

I had JoAnn Baldwin contact Grace right away, and a few days later, we were having the conversation I've just described.

I moved my chair out from behind the desk and closer to Grace, and I put my hand on her arm.

"I think Marnie's condition is operable," I said, "and if you agree, I'll schedule the surgery for tomorrow morning."

"Oh yes, please," and with that she dissolved into tears.

Grace didn't seem to be interested in many of the details. The preceding weeks had exhausted her. Now she was content just to learn that something would be done for Marnie, and that her daughter might get well.

Tania took Grace under her wing, making arrangements for her to stay at the Ronald MacDonald House, on East Eighty-sixth Street, which accommodates parents of seriously ill children who have come to New York for treatment.

The next day, I performed a craniotomy on Marnie and was able to resect most of the tumor. Marnie, with the great resilience of infants, came through the surgery with flying colors.

We followed up with a course of chemotherapy, under the direction of Jeff Allen. Grace was with Marnie constantly, comforting her when her stomach was upset, swaying her to sleep in her arms. All the time, Grace said little to the adults who cared for Marnie. Except for the phone calls she received from her husband every afternoon, she seemed to be in a world of her own, a world that consisted only of her and Marnie.

Late one afternoon, I asked Grace to join me in my office.

"Dr. Allen is very pleased with Marnie's progress," I said. "He thinks she will get well."

Grace smiled for the first time since I had met her.

"Is he sure about that?" she asked.

"We can never be sure, but we can be hopeful," I replied.

A cloud passed over her face, and then she seemed to hesitate to say more.

"It *is* good news," I stated emphatically.

"But the other doctor was pretty sure," she said with a touch of bitterness, "pretty sure that Marnie would die."

She was asking whether she could trust Jeff Allen and me after the medical system had failed her once.

Grace wasn't the only one who felt embittered by her experience. I did, too. Why, I asked myself, had she been so misinformed initially? What if her friend hadn't seen that television program?

A few weeks later, Grace and Marnie Brinn went home, with Marnie's prognosis declared to be good. Still, I remained haunted by what Grace's experience had been before she was able to see me.

If I had known Grace Brinn when Marnie first became ill, there are many things I would have told her. And now that I'm writing this book, at last I have the means of getting my message across to other parents, both those who suspect that their child is seriously ill and those who have already received a diagnosis.

Parents in the former category should trust their instincts and treat with skepticism any diagnosis that doesn't seem to jibe with what they know about their child's behavior. In particular, they should insist on having more tests performed.

Brain tumors, for example, are often difficult to diagnose because the symptoms can start off slowly. They also mimic other diseases. But if, over a period of time, a child experiences headaches that are worse just after wakening, vomits with or without nausea, becomes sluggish or drowsy, and shows a growing lack of coordination, an MRI and other diagnostic tests for tumor are needed.

Once a diagnosis of brain tumor or any other operable condition has been made, parents should insist on being referred to a surgeon who specializes in working with children. All too often a family doctor will automatically send the patient to a surgeon who is associated with his or her own institution, whether or not that person has particular expertise in operating on children.

Unfortunately, many primary physicians don't know that a whole range of pediatric surgical subspecialties—general surgery, neurosurgery, urology, ophthalmology, and cardiology— is now available. Others downplay the importance of these specializations, assuming that any qualified surgeon who operates on adults can also operate on children.

But experience counts in surgery, as it does in everything else. An auto mechanic who works only on transmissions undoubtedly repairs them better than one who spends most of his time on other types of repairs. A commercial airline pilot, unless he has special training, is not equipped to fly a fighter plane. Even though these analogies are simplistic, they are applicable to surgery, because children are not simply "little adults." They require the expertise of surgeons who can devote most of their time to them.

Parents must make certain that they have been referred to an appropriate surgeon. That means asking a question such as, "What proportion of your practice is devoted to children?" The answer should be: at least 60 percent. Parents should also find out about the surgeon's training, particularly how much of his or her residency was spent working with children. Another important question for parents to ask is: "Are you board certified?" (Information on certification can also be obtained from the American Board of Medical Specialties, 1–800–776–CERT.)

Parents often hesitate to ask questions, out of concern for the surgeon's feelings, but no doctor worthy of the name should resent these types of inquiries, especially at a time when people are in such distress.

Parents should try to evaluate the surgeon's personality, too. Does he or she seem to be an open person who will share information? Does the surgeon project a feeling of empathy? They'll be working with this doctor for a long time, so human qualities count for a great deal.

There's another important qualification: The surgeon chosen must be affiliated with a major medical center. Only such centers provide the type of care a seriously ill child needs: a team approach to care, including pediatricians, pediatric anesthesiologists, pediatric radiologists, and pediatric nurses; an excellent intensive care unit; and the availability of a pediatrician twenty-four hours a day.

In a large urban area, it's relatively easy to find a medical center by consulting the yellow pages or one of the medical schools in the vicinity. These schools are generally affiliated with medical centers, and a call to a department of neurosurgery can elicit the names of pediatric neurosurgeons who practice at a particular center.

If parents don't live in or near a city, there are several ways of locating the nearest medical center. One is to consult the *American Hospital Association Guide to the Health Care Field*, published annually and available at the public library. Another is to contact the state medical society.

The pediatric section of the American Association of Neurological Surgeons, 1-708-692-9500, can verify whether or not a specific pediatric neurosurgeon is a member of their organization. Other good sources are the American Brain Tumor Association, 3725 North Talman Avenue, Chicago, Illinois 60618, 1–800–886–2282, which keeps a list of physicians with a special interest in adult or pediatric brain tumor patients, and the Brain Tumor Foundation for Children, 751 DeKalb Industrial Way, Decatur, Georgia 30033, 1–404–458–5554.

As parents search for the best medical care, they must remember that having a seriously ill child makes them emotionally vulnerable. It's imperative for them to keep their judgment clear, and to be wary of anyone who claims to have a "cure" for cancer. There is no such thing. Though a parent can expect a doctor to provide a sense of hope and even optimism, one who promises to work miracles should be avoided.

Once parents have found the appropriate surgeon, it's essential to work closely with that person, to trust him or her completely, and to build toward an effective long-term relationship. Parents shouldn't be afraid to speak up, to share doubts and concerns, no matter how busy or "important" the surgeon seems to be. The doctor should be willing to make the necessary time to answer their questions and to be supportive.

It's also important that the parents protect their physical and mental energies by allowing relatives and friends to help care for the child as much as possible, and even by asking for such help if it's not offered. Too often, friends hesitate to "interfere," when, in fact, they would be pleased to help, if asked.

Caring for a seriously ill child can tear families apart or bring them closer together. The more support that parents can arrange—respite care, attendance at self-help groups, or time out to talk with friends and relatives—the more positive a difficult experience can become.

No one needs to be alone with a cataclysmic problem. Medical help is out there. So is assistance from other parents who have lived through the same thing. Every day, new advances are occurring in terms of research, training, and technology. There are many reasons, I think, to hope, and few to despair. Most of all, there is the sustaining love between parent and child, love that can endure the transformations of illness, and perhaps even grow from them.

I was reminded of that fact one evening a few months ago. The move to our new offices had just been completed, and weary as I was, I was taking a moment to unpack the one carton I had labeled PERSONAL. It was a little difficult to see because the only light in the office came from a lamp I had borrowed from the suite down the hall. The electricians had yet to install the new lighting I had ordered.

Flipping through a couple of photographs, I came across a letter I had forgotten about. It was from a mother whose child I had treated a few years previously. I read through it quickly and found a paragraph that I had underlined.

"In the midst of our struggle, we have found a kind of happiness, though I'm not sure I could say where that feeling comes from. But it is deep, far deeper than I could have imagined. And even though we go on living in the shadow of tragedy, our lives are, in a peculiar way, richer than they were before. Now I understand the truth, the nobility really, of all those sayings about the importance of fighting on and not giving up. Maybe our happiness has something to do with that."

Amen, I thought.

I put the letters back in the carton, and as I did so, there was a hesitant knock at the door.

The door opened and a couple stood there, the parents of a child Tania had just admitted to the hospital.

In the evening dusk and the poor lighting, it was difficult to make out their faces. Standing there, framed in the door-way, they could have been any of the hundreds of parents I had come to know so well over the years.

Their tension was apparent in the stiff way they held them-selves, as if even a moment of relaxation would cause them to fall apart. They walked toward me, hand in hand. I knew that they desperately wanted to hear what I had to say, yet wished just as desperately that they didn't have to know me at all.

I could feel myself opening up to them as their features became clearer and the hope in their eyes more distinct.

As I stood up to greet these new yet old acquaintances, I sensed the power of my mission growing within me. The weariness was gone, replaced by a kind of joy at having yet another chance to make a difference, to overcome a cosmic mischance.

"I'm Dr. Epstein," I said, holding out my hand. "I think I can help you."